THE
Natural
Healing
& Nutrition
ANNUAL
1994

THE
Natural
Healing
& Nutrition
ANNUAL
1994

Edited by Mark Bricklin, Editor,
***PREVENTION* Magazine,**
& Matthew Hoffman,
***PREVENTION* Magazine Health Books**

Rodale Press, Emmaus, Pennsylvania

_____ OUR MISSION _____

We publish books that empower people's lives.

_____ RODALE BOOKS _____

Contributors to
The Natural Healing and Nutrition Annual 1994

Writers: Pamela Boyer, Lisa Delaney, Barb Fritz, Lisa
 Gabor, Greg Gutfeld, Sara J. Henry, William LeGro,
 Mary Persian Nagle, Cathy Perlmutter, Jean
 Rogers, Marion Roach Smith, Maggie Spilner,
 Margo Trott, Susan Zarrow

Book and Cover Designer: Greg Imhoff
Layout Designer: Ayers/Johanek Publication Design
Associate Research Chief, _Prevention_ Magazine: Pamela Boyer
Office Manager: Roberta Mulliner
Office Personnel: Julie Kehs, Mary Lou Stephen

Contents

■   ■

Foods for Life

Slimming Secrets

Medical Breakthroughs

Contents

Especially for Women

Staying Fit

Nutrition and Health Updates

Contents

Fabulous Everyday Recipes

Beautiful You

Mind and Body

Young for Life

SUPPLEMENTS AND COMMON SENSE

Some of the reports in this book give accounts of the professional use of nutritional supplements. While food supplements are in general quite safe, some can be harmful if taken in very large amounts. Be especially careful not to take more than these commonsense daily limits:

Vitamin A	2,000 IU
Vitamin B_6	50 mg
Vitamin D	400 IU
Selenium	100 mcg

NOTICE

This book is intended as a reference volume only, not as a medical manual. The information given here is designed to help you make informed decisions about your health. It is not intended as a substitute for any treatment that may have been prescribed by your doctor. If you suspect that you have a medical problem, we urge you to seek competent medical help.

Introduction

■   ■

Good Health Is Ageless

In 1513, the Spanish explorer Juan Ponce de Leon set sail with three ships in search of the mythical Fountain of Youth. A drink from this fabulous fountain, legend had it, would instantly make an old person young.

Ponce de Leon failed, of course, but his quest for eternal youth lives on. In fact, scientists now believe they've found what he was looking for—not in old stories but in hard, scientific fact. There is increasing evidence that what today we might call future youth—measured in zest, mental energy and exuberant good health—can be achieved no matter what your chronological age. And you don't need to sail the globe to find it. The fountain—or font, if you will—is right here: the 1994 edition of *The Natural Healing and Nutrition Annual.*

In the last 12 months, we talked to scores of America's top scientists—cardiologists, rheumatologists, nutritionists and more—and asked them what we should be doing to look, feel and act as young as possible. They came through—with their top ten age erasers. We expected a trickle of information, but instead we got a flood. Some fountain!

The experts agreed that having a good diet belongs at or near the top of our list of age erasers. Research is accumulating fast that good nutrition can help restore verve and youthful good health. One study, for example, found that vitamin E—which is found in large amounts in green leafy vegetables—can reduce the risk for cataracts and heart disease.

In another study, people with high blood pressure were given a high-potassium diet. As a result, more than a third were able to stop taking their medication. How's that for turning back the clock? And while we're on the subject of blood pressure, another study found that people who lowered theirs had better sex than those stuck with higher numbers. Now that's a "side effect" we can live with!

Our quest didn't stop there. We also discovered that

in order to feel like a youngster, you have to *move* like one. That's where overall fitness comes in. A study found that older adults who took care of themselves—firemen and police officers, for example—performed just as well on the job as did their younger counterparts. By staying mentally and physically fit, the "seniors" were far snappier than their calendar years would suggest.

Overall fitness is also a big boost for people who have osteoarthritis. In one study, people who embarked on an exercise and therapy program had less pain and more strength after just three months. Other studies have shown that moderate exercise is good for your mental health, too. Better yet, you don't have to be a major league athlete to tap your body's supply of feel-good endorphins. Just taking a ten-minute brisk walk can get you started.

Of course, you can't feel young unless you also feel good. So we've included some of this year's most exciting medical breakthroughs—everything from healing with light to new strategies for managing arthritis. We also asked weight-loss experts for the latest in diet strategies. Their advice? Eat more. That's right: You can lose weight by eating more—if you make the right choices.

And for the first time ever, we have included several chapters that are "just for women"—intelligent, thoughtful discussions about health, beauty and much more. Learn to look great and feel great, no matter what your age.

As you will discover reading these pages, there is really nothing magical about eternal youth. The hard part (as poor Ponce de Leon found out) is finding the fountain. And you've already arrived!

Until next year . . .

The Editors
Prevention Magazine

Foods
for
Life

1 Skim Your Health Risks

An everyday remedy that's easy to swallow.

By George L. Blackburn, M.D., Ph.D.

Imagine if there were a natural substance that lowered cholesterol, without any unpleasant side effects. Imagine if the same substance helped keep bones and muscles strong, reduced fat and calories in the diet and maybe even brought down blood pressure. And imagine if this stuff were amazingly inexpensive, widely available and easy to swallow.

Well, this wonder substance exists, and you don't need a prescription for it. It's called skim milk.

Adult Americans don't get enough dairy products in general and enough skim milk in particular. Most nutritionists agree that nearly everyone (except infants) should consume at least two eight-ounce servings of dairy products daily. Americans generally take in less than half of that. Of all the dairy products available, skim milk, in my opinion, is the best choice. Why? Because it has the vitamin D and calcium needed for strong bones yet saves your daily fat ration for other uses. And I do mean *skim* milk—you really need to switch down from whole milk to 2 percent milk to 1 percent milk and then skim to enjoy the most health benefits.

Like other dairy products, *skim* milk is packed with nutrients. Yet, compared with other dairy products, skim milk contains virtually no fat and a minimum of calories, making it a super diet food. But the number-one reason to drink skim milk is for what we could call the "trickle-down" effect: A couple of glasses a day can improve your entire diet. Why? Because lactose, the dairy sugar in a glass of skim milk, is uniquely filling. Our experience has shown that when people drink more skim milk, they tend to eat less junk—less caffeine-containing beverages like coffee and tea; fewer sugary soft drinks; fewer sugary, calorie-laden foods and juices; less fat-heavy whole milk and other whole-milk dairy products.

If you want to reform your diet but are overwhelmed by all the changes that you've read are important, one excellent first step is to replace all beverages, including whole and low-fat milk products, with skim milk. You can save an amazing amount of fat. If most of the fat in your diet has come from dairy products, that first step may also be your last step: The switch to skim alone might reduce the amount of fat you eat to the target range recommended to prevent heart disease and certain cancers. (The goal is to bring total fat intake to around 25 percent of calories from fat; most Americans currently get about 37 percent of their calories from fat.)

The next big reason to drink fortified skim milk is for the calcium and vitamin D. These nutrients are critical for strong bones as well as other vital cell functions. This is particularly important for women of all ages, who are most susceptible to osteoporosis.

Another reason to drink skim milk is for the proteins and protein-related growth factors. Besides complete proteins (it has all the essential amino acids), milk contains special protein substances that promote growth and build and restore muscle—valuable for active people.

And finally, there's a growing body of research suggesting that skim milk may lower cholesterol and blood pressure. This new research is pointing toward a day when skim milk may be taken like a supplement or medication as a harmless, inexpensive way to control cholesterol.

The Cholesterol Connection

There are several studies showing a link between increased milk intake and lowered cholesterol. The latest evidence comes from a study conducted by researchers at Pennsylvania State University in University Park. During a one-week initial baseline period, researchers measured the cholesterol, blood pressure and triglycerides of 64 people aged 21 to 73. The researchers then asked these people to add a quart of solids-fortified skim milk to their daily diets.

Researchers continued to take the same measurements during the remaining eight weeks of the milk-supplementation experiment. Results of the comparison: Among the people whose cholesterol started at or above 190 milligrams per deciliter (mg/dl), cholesterol levels dropped dramatically, by 6.6 percent at the end of the eight weeks. Overall, for the entire group, cholesterol levels dropped 5.7 percent.

If 6 percent doesn't sound like much to you, consider this: Every 1 percent drop in cholesterol creates a 2 percent decline in coronary mortality.

Of course, not everyone who added skim milk enjoyed a cholesterol drop. People whose cholesterol was low to begin with (190 mg/dl or lower) didn't experience a change. Also, cholesterol levels didn't fall among people who were already on cholesterol-lowering medication.

Not surprisingly, the people who drank skim milk also wound up eating slightly less fat than they did before the study. The researchers noticed a 2 to 3 percent reduction in the percentage of calories from fat. How much did that have to do with the cholesterol drop?

Most of that reduction in fat intake didn't occur until after the largest fall in blood cholesterol, says lead researcher Gerald Buonopane, Ph.D., now consumer safety officer with the Food and Drug Administration. "So the fat reduction may have had some effect on cholesterol, but something else was going on."

That "something else," scientists suspect, has to do with the complex compounds in milk that we haven't yet fully identified. Cholesterol is produced in the liver through the action of several enzymes. Milk contains factors that may suppress production of those enzymes. One such factor that scientists have identified is called orotic acid. Dairy products contain small but potentially effective amounts of orotic acid.

In this study, scientists also found a relationship between increased skim milk consumption and reduced blood pressure. This may be partly related to the calcium and potassium in milk. But again, there may be unidentified substances involved.

Finally, the people in the study whose cholesterol levels started out high enjoyed significant reductions of nearly 12 percent in serum triglycerides, another risk factor for heart disease. Triglyceride levels didn't change for people who began with low cholesterol. The reason for a triglyceride connection isn't clear yet, and not all studies support a link to milk consumption. I theorize that if the triglyceride drop is real, it may be linked to a reduction in overall levels of sugar in the diet that occurred when people drank more skim milk.

Scientists can't say for sure that skim milk reliably lowers cholesterol, blood pressure and triglycerides. It does seem to help some people more than others. But we do know enough about skim milk that we can recommend it without hesitation for almost everyone, and especially people concerned about reducing fat in their diet and cholesterol in their blood.

Like the Benefits, Hate the Milk?

Some people dislike the taste and texture of skim milk. Some comments that are often heard: "It's too watery" and "It turns my coffee gray." But there are ways to improve both. Here are some ideas.

■ Exercise your blender. Get into skim-milk–based shakes, flavored with anything from vanilla or almond extract to frozen bananas or fresh raspberries. Sinfully good!

■ Look for skim milk that's fortified with milk solids (many brands on the market are). Or add several tablespoons of nonfat dry milk to every gallon of skim milk. It really thickens skim milk—your family may not even notice that you've switched from 1 percent or 2 percent milk to skim.

■ Try nonfat dry milk in your coffee or other hot beverage instead of liquid skim milk. Believe it or not, the dry stuff turns coffee the same warm brown color that cream creates.

For many people, the problem with skim milk has less to do with the taste on the tongue than with the turmoil in the tummy. Milk contains a complex sugar called lactose. Millions of people have trouble digesting milk because their gut doesn't produce adequate amounts of lactase, the enzyme that breaks up lactose. These people are "lactose intolerant."

But there are ways to get around lactose intolerance.

■ **Add cocoa.** Try cocoa-flavored skim-milk shakes, naturally sweetened with a banana or with a small amount of sweetener. Preliminary research suggests cocoa may reduce symptoms of lactose intolerance.

■ **Drink milk in small doses.** Drink four four-ounce glasses of skim milk daily instead of two eight-ounce glasses. Small amounts are easier to digest.

■ **Add skim milk to soups, baked goods and other recipes. And drink it with foods.** If it's consumed with fiber, the stomach takes longer to digest it and won't be so overwhelmed.

■ **Try lactase-enzyme supplements.** These supplements, often found in drugstores and health-food stores, split lactose molecules into easily digestible pieces. There's a liquid form that can be stirred directly into milk, without changing flavor or texture.

2   Packaged Prevention

For some people, vitamin and mineral supplements make good sense.

After a decade or so in which fats and cholesterol have hogged the spotlight of nutrition research, vitamins are making a big-time comeback. No matter where you look, there's a vitamin (or a mineral) surrounded by scientists saying "Aha!" A few examples:

■ A Harvard study found that supplements of beta-carotene taken by 165 male physicians with signs of heart disease reduced by one-half their number of strokes, heart attacks, cardiac deaths and artery-opening medical procedures, compared with a similar group of men not getting the supplements. The lucky group took a 50-milligram dose of beta-carotene (the amount found in two cups of cooked carrots) every other day for six years.

■ In another Harvard-associated study, nurses who, on their own, had been taking upwards of 100 international units of vitamin E a day were found to have 36 percent less risk of heart attack. (Eating lots of fruits and vegetables was found to cut risk by 22 percent, compared with women who ate few fruits and veggies.)

■ The British Medical Research Council discovered that supplements of folic acid, one of the B vitamins, apparently can prevent upwards of 70 percent of certain serious birth defects in children born to women with a known high risk. The supplement (four milligrams daily) had to be taken prior to conception.

■ Early, unconfirmed research shows that vitamin C intake of 180 milligrams per day (three times the Recommended Dietary Allowance—RDA—of 60 milligrams) was associated with higher HDL cholesterol, the protective part of cholesterol, it's reported from the USDA Human Nutrition Research Center on Aging at Tufts University in Boston.

■ In Latin American cancer centers, women who had the highest dietary intake of vitamin C and beta-carotene and other carotenoids (all found in fruits and vegetables) were found to have 30 to 40 percent less risk of developing cervical cancer.

And there are many other studies that add exciting dimensions to the possibility of added health protection by careful attention to vitamin intake.

Vitamin and Mineral Supplement Guidelines

Nutrient	RDA*	Protective Range
Vitamins		
Vitamin A†	5,000 IU	5,000 IU
Beta-carotene	6 mg‡	15-30 mg
Thiamine (B_1)	1.5 mg	1.5 mg
Riboflavin (B_2)	1.8 mg	1.8 mg
Niacin	20 mg	20 mg
Vitamin B_6	2 mg	2–10 mg
Vitamin B_{12}	2 mcg	2–10 mcg
Folate	200 mcg	400–800 mcg
Vitamin C	60 mg	100–500 mg
Vitamin D	10 mcg (400 IU)	10 mcg (400 IU)
Vitamin E	15 IU (10 mg αTE)	100–400 IU (67–268 mg αTE)
Minerals		
Calcium	1,200 mg	1,200–1,500 mg
Chromium§	50–200 mcg	100–200 mcg
Iron||	15 mg	15 mg
Magnesium	400 mg	400 mg
Selenium	70 mcg	70–100 mcg
Zinc	15 mg	15 mg

NOTES: Amounts listed here are in addition to nutrients obtained from food.

Don't take more than the upper limit of the Protective Range unless prescribed by a licensed health professional. Supplements are best taken with meals, particularly calcium, which needs the stomach acid produced by eating to enhance digestion.

*Represents the highest Recommended Dietary Allowances for all ages and sex groups except pregnant and lactating women.

†Vitamin A is best taken in the form of beta-carotene.

‡6 milligrams of beta-carotene provides 100 percent of the RDA for vitamin A.

§Range for chromium is an Estimated Safe and Adequate Daily Dietary Intake.

\|\|Men should not take supplemental iron without checking first with their doctors.

Supplemental Protection

It's sometimes said that we can get all the vitamins and minerals we need from ordinary foods. That's largely true. But it's also misleading.

If you are diligent in your nutritional habits, if you follow the ideas expressed in the recommendations of U.S. health and nutrition agencies, yes, you can do it. Women may have a hard time hitting the calcium and iron requirements, but it can be done.

Only it isn't. The latest survey of nearly 12,000 people shows that only 9 percent are eating the three or more daily servings of vegetables and two or more servings of fruits recommended by the U.S. Department of Agriculture and the Department of Health and Human Services. All those missing fruits and vegetables are exactly the major source of the protective nutrients— beta-carotene, vitamin C, vitamin E and folate.

When you consider that this poor showing comes after a major upsurge in consumption of fresh produce (broccoli, for instance), it's hard not to conclude that achieving the food consumption goals is at present beyond the grasp of most of us. Even many dietitians, surveys show, take nutritional supplements.

Certainly, the foundation of good nutrition is good food. There are key elements in food that simply aren't found in supplements or pills. Some of these are familiar, like fiber. But others, like siblings of beta-carotene and other compounds that may help prevent disease, are just now being studied. So food comes first.

Having done our best, though, we may feel it wise to fill in any gaps in our nutrition with supplements.

How Much Is Enough— But Safe?

The subject of nutritional supplements is inherently confusing—just like the rest of nutrition! Only your doctor or dietitian can make an intelligent recommendation as to what your individual needs are in food and nutrition.

What can be provided, though, are some broad guidelines on the amounts that may provide a good degree of potential protection without going overboard into unsafe overdoses.

The place to start a supplement program is with a good multiple. The problem, though, is that many multiples are needlessly high in some factors (B vitamins, for instance) while very low in others, like calcium—a mineral you need so much of that it simply won't fit into the average pill.

Choose a multiple that has the RDA of as many nutrients as possible. It's recommended that it contain vitamin A in the form of beta-carotene, which has more potential for chemoprevention and much less possibility of creating a harmful overdose.

Keep in mind that the RDA amounts of these nutrients are being added to what you're already eating in your food. So you're getting more than the "bare minimum."

Research is ongoing, so it's unclear whether supplementation above this level will prove to be of substantial benefit. For each nutrient, the table on page 8 shows a "protective range" of intake, which reflects amounts being used in much current research along with pertinent safety limits. In some cases the protective range is identical to the RDA. Remember, any supplementation regimen should be combined with your best efforts at a balanced diet.

3   Supermarket Makeovers

Fabulous new foods
with a fraction of the fat.

There's a quiet takeover under way in your local supermarket. Perhaps you haven't even noticed, but right there, in the dairy case and packaged-goods aisles, the rebels are assembling. Virtually indistinguishable from the mass of other products on the shelves, they have one thing in common that sets them apart from all others. They're fat free. Go ahead and taste them. Chances are, you too will defect (from those familiar high-fat prepared foods) and join the new fat-free revolution. You're certain to be glad you did.

Good News

We all know that a low-fat eating plan (along with a regular exercise regimen) is key to long-term weight control. But dietary programs can be quite a challenge over the long term. After all, until recently, adherence to a low-fat diet meant avoiding many of the foods we've grown to love. Now, thanks to a little food-processing ingenuity and a growing nutrition-conscious market, you can keep your fat intake in line without giving up the tastes you love!

Cookies, frozen desserts, puddings and a multitude of other popular foods have gone lean—really lean.

Think of the positive impact these foods can have on a heart-healthy diet, too. After all, many of the food products that have gone fat free were originally heavy in butter and cream—both major sources of saturated fat. And research indicates that fat, especially saturated fat (found mainly in animal products) drives up blood cholesterol. That's why lowering intake of overall fat and saturated fat has been strongly recommended by the National Cholesterol Education Program. It's also why the new fat-free alternatives come as welcome news to anyone who's cholesterol conscious.

Here are some of the new, low-fat foods on the market today.

Cheeses ▶ Cheeses can be one of the foods people find most difficult to give up in order to control cholesterol or lose weight. Whole-milk mozzarella has over six grams of total fat and nearly four grams of saturated fat per ounce. Cheddar is even more trouble, with over nine grams of total fat and almost six grams of saturated fat per ounce. Thanks to newer fat-free varieties, we can feel good about eating our cheesy favorites again. Alpine Lace Free N' Lean Cheddar was tested to see how it held up

11
∎

against a traditional cheese. Although there was a definite difference in texture and taste, the Alpine Lace was
not bad. Melted on top of a piece of toast with a slice of
tomato, it was quite good.

The nonfat mozzarella was voted an acceptable alternative to whole-milk mozzarella, too. And the Alpine
Lace nonfat cheddar has about 70 fewer calories than
traditional cheddar. That's a big savings in itself.

THE SECRET INGREDIENT: A GOOD WHIPPING

What makes the nonfat versions of foods so
similar to their fat-rich ancestors? The answer is they
feel like they have fat in them. That's not done by
bizarre and possibly risky new chemicals, either.
What does the trick is novel manipulation of many
familiar ingredients.

"One fat replacement, Simplesse, is made from
proteins that are microparticulated, or beaten into
tiny spheres," says Rudolph Harris, Ph.D., consumer
safety officer for the Food and Drug Administration.
"These particles are so small that when they are put
into a food in place of fat, the product actually has
the feel of a fat to the mouth."

Simplesse is the fat substitute in Simple Pleasures, the frozen dairy dessert that was tested. It is
made from microparticulated egg whites and/or milk
proteins and other ingredients.

Many of the other fat replacements in fat-free
and low-fat products are the result of commercial
techniques of acidifying, blending or heating proteins,
carbohydrates or fat-based ingredients. Common food
ingredients like gums, pectin and starches are used.
Other fat replacements that are just as standard as
other natural ingredients are dextrin, polydextrose,
maltodextrin and cellulose. The innovative use of
these elements in foods is recognized as acceptable by
the American Dietetic Association.

12

Cookies ▶ Remember Mom's homemade oatmeal cookies? Even today, most recipes call for a stick or two of butter for a batch. Not surprisingly, then, each cookie can ooze with 2 grams of fat, over ½ gram of it saturated fat. Switch to Frookie's fat-free oatmeal-raisin version (which tasters found to be quite tasty and chewy) and you're in for big fat savings—4 grams for a two-cookie snack.

You can find other varieties of fat-free cookies as well. Health Valley, for example, offers a wide selection of nonfat cookies and fruit bars.

Crackers ▶ Wheat crackers are not high-fat demons if you eat a modest number of them. Modesty, unfortunately, is not always snacking policy. At about 60 calories a serving (that's just seven crackers), wheat crackers also deliver almost two grams of total fat, one gram of it saturated.

Health Valley to the rescue again. They've come out with a line of fat-free crackers that are terrific for snacking with your favorite low-fat and nonfat dips. The Organic Wheat with Natural Herbs flavor is quite good. And they have 20 fewer calories and over twice the fiber of ordinary wheat crackers. Although they are a bit dry when eaten plain, these crackers have a distinct flavor that would easily complement salsa or a low-fat bean dip.

Cream Cheese ▶ Alpine Lace has done it again. Their new Free N' Lean Fat Free cream cheese and cream-cheese spreads boast a trim 4 percent of calories from fat—compared to ordinary cream cheese with 90 percent fat calories. (Although Free N' Lean isn't completely fat free, each serving contains less than ½ gram of fat.) You save 10 grams of fat (over 6 grams of it saturated fat) and about 70 calories with every ounce (two tablespoons).

Alpine Lace Free N' Lean Fat Free cream-cheese spreads come in many tempting flavors. You can choose from garlic and herb, cheddar cheese, cheddar cheese with jalapeño, and cream cheese and chive flavors. So, spread the news—cream cheese has gone fat free!

13

Egg Substitutes ▶ The little guys look harmless enough. But eggs contain 5 grams of total fat—over 1½ grams of it saturated—and 75 calories each. Frozen egg substitutes are now available fat free and have cut out two-thirds of the calories from the real McCoy. Although they aren't the newest fat-free foods available, the variety of uses for egg substitutes establishes them as a universal kitchen staple.

Frozen Desserts ▶ Simple Pleasures—the name does not deceive you. This nonfat frozen dairy dessert tastes delightful and has a smooth, creamy consistency. With products like this, you'll never scream for ice cream again! In fact, the only discernible difference detected by tasters was that it did not coat the tongue and linger the way ice cream does. But, hey, when you consider the fat savings (almost 7½ grams of saturated fat and nearly 12 grams of total fat per ½-cup serving) compared with premium vanilla ice cream, you'll agree it's a winning choice.

Many nonfat frozen yogurts have also appeared on the market in recent years and are quite delicious. By substituting nonfat vanilla yogurt for a ½-cup serving of premium vanilla ice cream, you save about 12 grams of fat—7½ grams of it saturated—and are spared about 75 calories.

Granola Bars ▶ This ever-popular snack food is usually only moderately high in fat, although some brands do contain more as a result of high-fat additions such as chocolate chips.

Once again, Health Valley has come up with a palatable fat-free snack. Their granola bar saves you almost 8½ grams of fat (over 1 gram of saturated) when compared with an ordinary bar the same size. And let's not overlook the almost 80 calories you save as well.

Mayonnaise-Style Dressing ▶ Kraft Free has done it. They have created a terrific nonfat mayonnaise-style dressing. When blended into tuna, chicken or potato salad, it is virtually indistinguishable from the traditional oil-laden versions. Each tablespoon saves you 11 grams of fat, and over 1½ grams of it is saturated fat.

14

Muffins ▶ Great any time of day, muffins can be a terrific source of fiber. Butter, oil and other high-fat ingredients, however, make many of them undesirable. McDonald's (yes, the golden arches) has come up with a fat-free apple-bran muffin that is perfect for people on the go. A traditional homemade muffin the same size has almost 8 grams of total fat, with almost 2½ grams of it saturated fat.

Health Valley has also created a few varieties of fat-free muffins, available in your supermarket or health-food store. The muffins come in flavors like banana, apple-raisin and raisin-spice. Compared with a like-size, traditional bran muffin, a Health Valley fat-free muffin saves over 5 grams of total fat and 1½ grams of saturated fat.

Pudding ▶ Traditional chocolate pudding is a favorite dessert for many people. But with 6 grams of fat per serving (almost 3½ grams of which are saturated fat), that's a far cry from a light dessert.

Now, however, there's a pudding that's just as delightful and creamy as any pudding you've ever tasted—and (you guessed it) it's fat free. Tasters who tested Jell-O Free Chocolate-Vanilla Swirl Pudding Snacks, available in serving-size cups in the dairy case, gave it a "thumbs up." The consistency and flavor were as good as original Jell-O Pudding Snacks. Of course, fat-wise and calorie-wise, the Jell-O Free Pudding Snacks were a hit, too. Compared with the original version, they were 70 calories lighter; compared with homemade, they had about 90 fewer calories.

You can also buy instant pudding mixes in various flavors and make your own fat-free dessert by using skim milk instead of whole milk or low-fat (1 or 2 percent) milk.

Sour Cream ▶ Yikes! Regular sour cream has three grams of fat (almost two grams of it saturated) in every tablespoon. Thank goodness for fat-free sour creams. Not only do they eliminate the fat, they are also about 20 calories lighter per tablespoon. Tasters who tried Light

N' Lively brand found it satisfying. Nonfat sour cream is a great way to keep Mexican dishes and baked potatoes from becoming cholesterol nightmares. It also holds up well in cooking.

4   If You Can't Eat 'Em, Juice 'Em!

A complete guide to juices and juicers.

Did you eat your health quota of fruits and vegetables today? The National Center for Health Statistics notes that very few Americans did. For whatever reason, only 9 percent manage to chow down the bare minimum of five servings a day (as recommended by the U. S. Department of Agriculture). Even the most health-minded among us may have difficulty swallowing the seven to nine servings per day that many nutrition experts say is optimum.

No wonder people have taken to the glad refrain: If you can't eat 'em, juice 'em.

Fresh fruits and vegetables are really worth their weight in good health! Studies have repeatedly shown that when more produce is consumed, less cancer occurs. And less heart disease, less hypertension, less cataracts, less diabetes and fewer weight problems.

What's the connection? Most fruits and vegetables are nearly fat free and chock-full of fiber. Plus, their unique combination of vitamins, minerals and other food factors, scientists say, contributes to their cancer-fighting potential. Beta-carotene, a vitamin found exclusively in fruits and vegetables—chiefly in deep green and orange-fleshed varieties—is among the rising stars in nutritional research. Diets high in beta-carotene–rich foods have shown promise in preventing heart disease as well as certain kinds of cancer.

Fruits and vegetables are so healthful in part

because they have lots of dietary fiber. Fresh, unsweet-ened fruit or vegetable juice usually has very little fiber. But it's a powerhouse of nutrients—sort of a vitamin-and-mineral supplement in a glass.

Supplements in a Glass

Drinking vegetable and fruit juice is a great way to "supplement" your diet with vitamins, minerals and other phytochemicals (naturally occurring chemical substances present in plants) that help prevent cancer. You'd have to chew your way through six good-size carrots to get the beta-carotene in one easy-to-swallow eight-ounce glass of freshly extracted carrot juice. (Fresh, homemade juices do have a slight advantage over commercial varieties: Many commercial juices are heat processed and stored for long periods, which can diminish nutritional values.)

From a weight-watcher's standpoint, vegetable juice is just what the doctor ordered. Fat-wise and calorie-wise, it's practically a freebie. That makes it a smart alternative to sugary soft drinks. And consid-ering its hefty dose of vitamins and minerals, vegetable juice is arguably even a better beverage choice than water.

The Fiber Facts

What juice gains in concentration of nutrients, however, it usually loses in fiber. An eight-ounce glass of extracted carrot juice contains a scant 2 grams of fiber, compared with 14 grams in the six large carrots (one pound) it takes to make it. Keeping in mind fiber's important role in lowering cholesterol, preventing cancer and taming appetites, nutrition experts warn that extracted juice should be considered a supplement to, not a replacement for, fiber-rich foods.

Another caveat, notes Kathryn Miller, R.D., of the Cooper Center for Aerobics Research in Dallas, is that fruit juice is a concentrated source of fructose, a natural sugar, and can deliver quite a caloric punch. (At about

112 calories per eight-ounce glass, apple juice is equivalent to cola, which contains from 103 to 114 calories.)

People with blood sugar problems like diabetes need to be especially cautious. All that sugar in juices—and little fiber to slow its absorption—can send blood sugar levels soaring. For this reason, you may want to use sugar-free beverages like sparkling water to dilute the fruit juice.

Home Juicing

And let's not forget about the joy of juicing. Selecting and juicing your produce fresh from the market or roadside stand can be as delightful as drinking the "fruits" of your efforts.

Because juicing requires practically no prep work—most produce needs only to be rinsed and cut into chunks—the biggest challenge may be deciding which juicer to invest in. While home juicers can be had for $120, many well-built models run as high as $300 or more. So, weigh your purchase carefully. Then, have fun.

For starters, try some of the vitamin-, mineral- and energy-packed recipes that follow. Each of the recipes can be made using either a juice extractor or a Vita-Mix (blender-type) juicer. When creating these drinks or experimenting on your own, be sure to read and follow manufacturers' directions carefully. For maximum freshness, keep your raw ingredients cold until ready to use. Serve juices over ice or at room temperature, according to your taste.

Melon Wakeup

Start your day with a breakfast juice power-packed with beta-carotene and vitamin C. If you prefer a tarter juice, substitute one-half grapefruit for the orange. This juice can be converted to a melon spritzer simply by topping it off with sparkling water.

¼ medium cantaloupe
1 medium orange
½ cup watermelon chunks
Lime juice

Slice the cantaloupe flesh away from the rind and cut into chunks. Peel and section the orange, leaving some of the pithy white area.

Process all ingredients. Add a spritz of lime juice and serve.

Makes 1⅓ cups

Blackberry Borscht
Rich, dark, pulpy and dramatic, this sweet/tart blend could pass for soup. It's like drinking a meal, so take it slow.

    2 medium carrots
    1 medium beet with tops
    ½ cup blackberries
    ¼ medium cantaloupe
       Lemon juice

Wash the carrots and remove peels. Wash the beet and tops, then remove the tops so they can be fed into the juicer easily.

Rinse the blackberries. Slice the cantaloupe flesh away from the rind and cut into chunks.

Process all ingredients. Add a spritz of lemon juice and serve chilled or over ice.

Makes 1½ cups

Ginger Fizz
High in beta-carotene and potassium, this all-around favorite may even soothe a tummyache with its little zinger of ginger.

    2 medium carrots
    ½ small bunch parsley
    ¼ small pineapple
    1 piece (½") fresh ginger

Wash the carrots and remove peels. Rinse the parsley and shake off water.

Cut the pineapple away from the skin and slice into spears.

Process all ingredients.

Makes 1 cup

Emerald Essence
A delicious, sparkling green, cocktail-type juice.

    4 leaves kale
    2 medium celery stalks, with leaves
    ¼ medium pineapple
       Mint sprigs (optional)

Wash the kale and celery. Cut the pineapple away from the skin and slice into spears.

Process all ingredients. Pour over ice and garnish with mint sprigs.

Makes 1 cup

High Energizer
Adapted from the Vita-Mix recipe booklet, this total-juice smoothie is designed to give you a healthy spurt of energy.

    ½ cup pineapple chunks
    ½ medium orange, peeled and seeded
    ½ ripe banana, peeled
    ½ cup strawberries
    1 slice (1") apple
    ¼ teaspoon cinnamon
    ½ cup ice

Place the ingredients in the juicer container in the order listed. Clamp the dome lid in place and process 1 minute or until smooth.

Makes 1½ cups

Veggie Vigor
The ultimate vegetable juice cocktail. Actually, it's a salad in a glass, only better! It's powerful, so be prepared.

    2 medium tomatoes
    2 medium carrots
    2 medium leaves kale
    2 medium leaves spinach
    1 medium celery stalk, with leaves
    ⅛ head cabbage (about ¼ lb.)
    1 piece (½") daikon radish
       Lemon juice

Rinse the tomatoes and cut into wedges. Wash the carrots and remove peels.

Wash the kale, spinach and celery. Wash the cabbage and cut into wedges.

Process all ingredients. Stir and add a spritz of lemon juice.

Makes 1½ cups

Carrot-Apple Gusto

A powerful, sweet concoction loaded with everything good. Another glassful of salad—this time Waldorf!

2 medium carrots
1 celery stalk
1 medium apple
1 medium beet with tops
1 cup parsley, loosely packed

Wash the carrots and remove peels. Wash the celery and apple and cut the apple into chunks.

Wash the beet and tops, then remove the tops so they can be fed into the juicer easily. Rinse the parsley and shake off water.

Process all ingredients.

Makes 1 cup

Three Juicers Compared

Before purchasing your juicer, you should know that there are two distinctly different methods of making juice. One is to puree the whole fruits and vegetables—pulp, rind, seeds and all. The other method is to grate the fruits and vegetables, then extract the juice from the pulp.

For pureeing fruits and vegetables, one machine stands head and motor above the rest: Vita-Mix. For juice extracting, there are many models, which operate either by hydraulic pump or centrifugal force. To compare the basic types of juicers—the super-powerful blender-type juicer and two juice extractors (one that uses a hydraulic pump and another that uses centrifugal force)—testers at *Prevention* magazine conducted an informal demonstration and taste test.

Three of the top juicers on the market were tested: Vita-Mix, Champion and Omega. Each juicer was tested, following manufacturers' directions, three separate times. Foods of distinctly different densities—carrots, pineapples and tomatoes—were used, and testers also noted each juicer's ease of assembly, operation and cleanup. Here's what they found.

Vita-Mix

Method of operation: A super-high-powered blender-type appliance that can puree whole fruits and vegetables (skin, seeds and all). It utilizes flat "hammermill" blades that, according to the manufacturer, "never need to be sharpened or replaced."

Assembly: Requires practically no assembly. Parts consist of a base, a blenderlike container and a see-through dome-shaped lid with built-in feeding tube. The lid clamps on easily.

Performance: Especially good for "juicing" soft- or medium-fleshed fruits, producing smooth drinks chock-full of all the fruit's original goodness and fiber. The tomatoes liquefied into a very flavorful and full-bodied juice, with a thick, souplike consistency. Simmering over medium heat for five to ten minutes, as the manufacturer suggests, does thin the juice, but our testers felt it destroyed some of the natural tomato flavor.

The pineapple juice was incredible! We mixed 2½ cups of fresh pineapple chunks with 1 cup of ice cubes, as the manufacturer directed. The result was a thick, sweet, creamy, frothy texture, like a tropical cocktail. Hard, fibrous vegetables, however, do not give up their essence as easily to the Vita-Mix—as we discovered when making carrot juice. Pureeing carrots wasn't the problem; the Vita-Mix rose to the challenge. But it was necessary to strain the carrot puree. We used a colander lined with cheesecloth. After pressing and squeezing the puree, we were able to extract a very smooth, sweet juice with a pure and good carrot flavor. The entire process took about five minutes.

Other uses: The most versatile of the juicers we

tested, a Vita-Mix can do anything a blender does—and more. It grinds grain and kneads dough, and it can whip up frozen desserts with or without yogurt.

Cleanup: Couldn't be easier. Simply fill with hot, soapy water and turn on. Or rinse the blenderlike container and dome-shaped lid and drain. And if that's too much trouble, just put the Vita-Mix in your dishwasher. Don't forget to flush the spout, since debris does collect there.

Buying information: For information on ordering, write to Vita-Mix Corp., Dept. PR0193, 8615 Usher Rd., Cleveland, OH 44138, or call (800) VITAMIX.

Champion

Method of operation: A juice extractor that finely chews the food, then extrudes the juice from the pulp using hydraulic pressure.

Assembly: Not difficult. Four to five separate pieces need to be assembled each time you juice, but after you've done it several times, the procedure becomes comfortable and easy. And the accompanying manual provides easy-to-understand instructions. You must supply your own bowls to collect the juice and pulp.

Performance: The Champion tackled each food with ease, usually producing a smooth and satisfying juice with some body to it. The carrot juice was especially full-bodied, even pulpy—a consistency one of our testers described as "good and hearty." The tomato juice was likewise rich-tasting—much thicker than store-bought juice. It also produced a fresh-looking product when compared with canned. The overall consensus of our testers was that it was "very good" to "excellent." Pineapple juice was the exception. The juice was thin, like store-bought pineapple juice. It did, however, have a very fresh pineapple flavor.

Other uses: The Champion comes with just one alternate attachment—a metal plate that fits over the juice filter. This plate prevents the juice from being extracted, resulting in a fine puree of fruit or vegetable. By feeding frozen fruit into the juicer fitted with this attachment, you can create fabulous soft-serve frozen-fruit desserts with no fat or sugar added. We tried it with frozen strawberries and in less than a minute, a rich, deep-red, smooth, refreshing confection appeared. An unsurpassed strawberry sorbet! Using this attachment, you can also grind grains.

Cleanup: All parts must be dismantled from the base and washed in cold, soapy water after each use. Not dishwasher-safe; parts sometimes stain but can easily be cleaned with a bleach solution.

Buying information: For information on ordering, write to Plastaket Manufacturing Co., Inc., 6220 E. Highway 12 (Victor Rd.), Lodi, CA 95240, or call (209) 369-4638.

Omega

Method of operation: Grates foods, then extracts the juice by centrifugal force. Fruits or vegetables are pressed against a rotating wheel of fine blades at the base of a sievelike basket. The grated produce is flung against the sieve. Juice filters through.

Assembly: Not difficult: The bowl fits into the base housing, and a strainer basket, blade and clutch nut fit into the bowl. The lid is clamped on with two side-latch arms, much like those on a foot locker.

Performance: Produced what many would consider the "perfect" carrot juice—rich-tasting with a beautiful orange color and a thick, slightly grainy "mouthfeel." One tester described it as "creamy-rich with a true carrot flavor."

Likewise, the pineapple juice drew "excellent" ratings from our tasters, who described it as smooth and frothy, full of the flavor of fresh pineapple.

Only the tomato juice proved slightly disappointing—too thick and frothy, according to our testers.

Other uses: Like other centrifugal-type juicers, the Omega does not come with attachments. It is designed exclusively for juice extraction.

Cleanup: Involves unscrewing the clutch nut that holds the blade and dismantling the pulp-catching cylindrical strainer from the bowl. The pulp must be scraped out by hand. (To facilitate this cleaning operation, paper filters, available from the manufacturer, can be inserted in the strainer before use.) The bowl, basket and blade parts should be rinsed with cool water—never with hot water and never in a dishwasher.

Buying information: For information on ordering, write to Omega Products, Inc., 6291 Lyters Ln., P.O. Box 4523, Harrisburg, PA 17111, or call (717) 561-1105.

Slimming
Secrets

Stave Off Food Cravings

5

Ten easy ways to keep your appetite under control.

Like an unruly child, your appetite sometimes throws a tantrum and demands more food. Against all reason, the cravings may even hit right after a large steak dinner. Or right out of nowhere.

Is there any rhyme or reason to these cravings? Scientists say yes. They've discovered that our appetites do indeed follow some underlying rules. Appetite, they say, is turned on both by what's happening outside of us—like whether someone's just offered us a doughnut— and what's happening inside our bodies—the biochemical signals between mouth, stomach, nervous system and brain. In one of the hottest new areas of research, scientists are discovering that certain foods may even trigger the desire to eat more, while other foods tend to suppress that desire.

New research points to at least ten different ways you can control the urge to eat, whenever or wherever it strikes you.

1. Drown Your Appetite ▶ "Drinking generous amounts of water is overwhelmingly the number-one way to reduce appetite," says George L. Blackburn, M.D., Ph.D., associate professor at Harvard Medical School and chief of the Nutrition/Metabolism Laboratory with the Cancer Research Institute at New England Deaconess Hospital in Boston. The reason: A lot of water takes up a lot of room in the stomach. The stomach feels full, reducing the desire to eat.

Water can quell the appetite in other ways. "Many people think they're having a food craving, when in fact they're thirsty," says Dr. Blackburn. So next time you get the urge to eat, try a cup of water instead.

Aim for 64 ounces of fluids daily. Don't gulp down an

entire glass at a time, as if it were medicine, or you'll never continue. Instead, sip 3 to 4 ounces at a time throughout the day.

2. Graze Sensibly ▶ Mom always warned us not to snack before mealtime to avoid ruining our appetite. But nowadays, scientists are rethinking Mom's advice.

Grazing means nibbling small amounts of food frequently, instead of eating just one to three large meals a day. Scientists who endorse it say grazing can keep your appetite down all day long and prevent bingeing.

James Kenney, R.D., Ph.D., nutrition research specialist at the Pritikin Longevity Center in Santa Monica, California, believes that grazing quashes the appetite because it keeps insulin levels steadier—and lower—than eating a few large meals.

A large meal, especially one that's sugary and high in fat, stimulates the body to produce lots of insulin. Its job: to remove all of those excess sugars and block the release of fats into the bloodstream.

Smaller, more frequent meals, on the other hand, keep insulin and blood sugar levels more stable, so the brain doesn't signal an urgent need for more fuel.

But for grazing to be effective, Dr. Kenney warns, you have to munch the right kinds of foods. "You cannot graze on M&M's, potato chips and Häagen-Dazs. Your insulin levels and appetite increase. But if you graze on low-fat, high-fiber foods that aren't packed with calories—like carrots, peaches, oranges, red peppers, pasta, potatoes or oatmeal—you keep your appetite down."

If grazing feels like too much freedom to eat, it may be helpful to schedule your grazing in advance. Plan to eat every two hours or so. Take your healthy goodies to work with you, so you aren't tempted by fattening fare.

3. Soup It Up ▶ A lot of research over the years suggests that soup has the ability to turn off the appetite with far fewer calories than many other foods.

In a study at Johns Hopkins University in Baltimore, researchers compared soup with other appetizers to see which most effectively dimmed the desire to eat. They invited 12 men to lunch every day for two weeks. On different days, the men received different appetizers: tomato soup, Muenster cheese on crackers, or fresh fruit. Calories in each appetizer portion were equal. Then the men were given a main course to eat.

The results: Tomato soup was the most satisfying appetizer. It beat out all the others in reducing the number of calories of the entrée that were consumed. The least satisfying appetizer was cheese and crackers. The soup reduced later calorie intake by 25 percent compared with cheese and crackers.

The researchers aren't sure just why soup is so satiating. In other tests, they found it wasn't the warmth of soup or the salt that made a difference; cold, less salty soup reduced appetite about as well. The key may be the large volume of space soup takes up in the stomach. Also, most of soup's calories come from carbohydrates rather than fat, and carbohydrates are more satisfying to the brain.

There may be a psychological factor as well, notes Dr. Kenney: "Hot soup is very relaxing if you have a nervous, gnawing appetite."

4. Eat More Complex Carbohydrates ▶ A few years ago, potatoes and pasta were forbidden foods among dieters. We were encouraged to dine on a hamburger (without the roll), with a side order of cottage cheese (nestled on a lettuce leaf).

Since then, high-protein, low-carbohydrate schemes have been debunked as unhealthy, ineffective in the long run and even potentially dangerous. Foods like rice, potatoes, corn and pasta that are high in complex carbohydrates and low in fat have made a big comeback. Among their many virtues for weight watchers is their powerful ability to satisfy the appetite with fewer calories.

Scientists offer a variety of fascinating theories to explain the appetite-quenching effect of foods that are high in carbohydrate and low in fat.

One hypothesis has to do with our body's primary fuel source, glycogen, a form of carbohydrate stored

29

mostly in the liver and muscles. The body can store only a couple of thousand calories of glycogen at a time, compared with over 100,000 calories that can be stored as fat.

High-fat foods don't switch off the "eat" message as effectively as foods that are high in carbohydrates, says Dr. Kenney. That's because dietary fat cannot be converted into glycogen, and glycogen (particularly that stored in the liver) appears to trigger the hunger signal to turn off.

Carbohydrates, on the other hand, are quickly converted to glycogen, so they shut the hunger signal off more quickly. For example, take one ounce of potato chips versus a whole baked potato. Each has 160 calories, but which is more likely to fill you up? Obviously, you end up eating a lot more calories from potato chips, loaded with fat, than from a baked spud (whose calories come primarily from carbohydrates) before you feel satisfied.

Additionally, if those carbohydrates are derived from whole grains, fruits, vegetables and beans instead of overprocessed sugars and starches, they refuel glycogen levels without overstimulating insulin levels.

What's more, Dr. Kenney adds, carbohydrates are digested and stored less efficiently than fat. "That means the metabolic rate goes up more when the body is metabolizing carbohydrates than when it's metabolizing fat. A higher metabolic rate produces more body heat, which is associated with reduced appetite. And according to my theory, whatever heats you up, slims you down."

There's yet another theory about why carbohydrates dim the appetite. It has to do with the connection between carbohydrates and the brain chemical serotonin.

Serotonin is a mood enhancer, and a lack of serotonin is linked with depression. The fact that many depressed people are also overweight has led some scientists to investigate the possibility that lack of serotonin stimulates food cravings, while boosting serotonin levels reduces appetite. They've discovered that carbohydrates seem to increase brain levels of serotonin—and reduce appetite. But this research is still in the early stages, says Thomas Wadden, Ph.D., director of the Center for Health Behavior at Syracuse University in New York.

Whatever the reason for carbohydrate's satisfying effects, it works. Nutritionists recommend 6 to 11 daily servings of grains like bread, cereal and pasta. It may take about 20 minutes from the time you eat a complex carbohydrate until the hypothalamus turns off your appetite. So if you're going out to dinner and are concerned that you may overeat, try a high-carbohydrate, low-fat "preload" about 20 minutes before the rest of the meal. Order whole-wheat bread (without the butter), soup with noodles or rice, or even a small serving of spaghetti. You'll wind up eating less food.

5. Say Yes to Spicy Foods ▶ Have you ever binged on a huge plate of spicy food—such as Mexican, Thai, Szechuan or Indian fare? It's nearly impossible. Those foods seem to quiet the appetite better than blander fare. One possible reason: "The flavor is so intense that we don't need as much," says Maria Simonson, Ph.D., Sc.D., director of the Health, Weight and Stress Clinic at Johns Hopkins Medical Institutions in Baltimore.

Spicy foods also speed the metabolism, says Dr. Kenney. "When people eat hot chili, they often sweat, a sure sign of increased metabolic rate. And the faster the metabolic rate, the more heat produced by the body. Remember, whatever warms you up, in turn slims you down."

So stock up on hot peppers, horseradish, chili powder and the like. Learn to use them often, especially in place of salt. "Salt does make some people eat more, perhaps by upping insulin levels," says Dr. Kenney. "But the best reason to avoid salt is because its use often leads to high blood pressure."

6. Feast on Fiber ▶ How does fiber satisfy? In many ways. Satisfaction begins in the mouth, and fibrous foods provide robust mouthfuls that must be chewed thoroughly. It's a natural way to slow down eating, and eating slower means eating less—the extra time lets the body know it's received fuel and doesn't need much more.

Next, fiber takes up a lot of room in the stomach, and increased stomach volume has been shown to reduce

31

appetite. So the stomach feels full longer.

Soluble fiber, best known for its cholesterol-cutting abilities, also dampens insulin response. Normally after a meal, insulin levels rise to help metabolize sugar and fat. But soluble fiber keeps insulin levels lower after a meal, says Dr. Kenney. The richest sources of soluble fiber include barley, oat products, beans, apples, citrus fruits and root vegetables like beets, carrots and potatoes.

Finally, foods that are high in fiber tend to have fewer calories in every bite, which means fewer calories consumed overall. Research at the University of Alabama shows that people eat many fewer calories on a low-calorie-density diet than on a high one, says Dr. Kenney.

Americans consume only about 12 to 15 grams of fiber daily, while 25 grams or more is recommended. Get fiber through food and not through fiber supplements; some are fraudulent, and others, if abused, can lead to severe constipation.

7. Eat Simply ▶ Your daughter-in-law has invited you to dinner and she's eager to please. There's freshly baked bread, a shrimp appetizer, a roast beef entrée, a potato side dish, rice pilaf, noodles, fresh corn, broccoli, raspberry pie, chocolate truffles and frozen yogurt.

If you're like most mortals, you'll want to try a little of everything. Unfortunately, by the end of the meal, that may translate into a lot of food.

Now imagine this: Instead of the multicourse feast, she serves a simple dinner of salad and a one-pot chicken-and-rice casserole, with raspberry pie for dessert. How likely is it that you'll overeat? Much less. "Serving a wide variety of foods at one meal can cause you to eat much more," says Dr. Wadden. "That's because each different food has its own satiety level." So after you've had as much shrimp as you want, you might still crave the roast beef. After the bread, you'll still want to try the potatoes, noodles and rice. And of course, it's nearly impossible to resist "just a taste" of every dessert.

So limit entrées and side dishes to one each at every meal. And look for some one-pot meals that your family can enjoy.

FOOD CRAVINGS:
RIDE THE WAVE

You're sitting at your desk, concentrating hard on your work, when suddenly an image seizes control of your brain. Carrot cake! You can taste it; you can smell it; you have to have it!

Sound familiar? Whether the yearning is for carrot cake, kosher pickles or chocolate-covered cherries, everyone has experienced a food craving at some time. "Food cravings are a normal part of living in a food-oriented society," says Linda Crawford, an eating-behavior specialist at Green Mountain at Fox Run, a residential weight- and health-management center for women in Ludlow, Vermont.

The problem, notes Crawford, is that many people interpret food cravings as commands. "People believe that cravings keep getting stronger, until they finally have to give in."

But in fact, research by G. Alan Marlatt, Ph.D., of the University of Washington in Seattle, shows that cravings follow more of a wave pattern. The craving starts and escalates, but then it peaks and subsides. "People need to know that it will decline," says Crawford. "When a food craving strikes, they might imagine themselves like a surfer. They have to ride that wave till it finally vanishes."

It's much easier to ride the wave if you distract yourself, Crawford says. "Ideally, you should do something incompatible with eating, like taking a walk." Give yourself 20 minutes to wait it out, she advises. "In 20 minutes, reevaluate the situation. The craving has probably diminished. Now what are you going to do about it? You can more rationally decide what, if anything, you're going to eat and how much of it you'll eat." As in surfing, practice makes perfect, adds Crawford. "The more you practice riding a wave, the easier it becomes."

8. Outbike Your Appetite ▶ Got the munchies? If you've tried a glass of water or a high-carbohydrate, high-fiber snack but they didn't do the trick, take a walk, ride an exercise bike or do some other activity.

Regular exercise reduces the appetite, in part by modifying the insulin response, which reduces the upward spike that has been associated with increased appetite. Exercise helps control blood sugar, leading to a steady state associated with fullness. Aerobic exercise reduces the appetite in the short run, says Dr. Kenney, perhaps because it heats the body. Not many people can eat a lot after exercise.

In the long run, a regular exercise program increases appetite somewhat. That's because you burn up your glycogen stores more quickly. This partially offsets the appetite-dimming effects of the temperature rise, says Dr. Kenney. But when you step up exercise, you usually don't eat quite enough calories to make up for the amount of fat you've burned off. Provided you're on a high-carbohydrate diet, you can replenish your glycogen stores without replacing the fat you burned off exercising.

Here's an example. Say you eat 1,600 calories a day but burn only 1,500. Over the long run, those hundred extra calories a day turn into extra pounds. But then you begin a daily exercise program. It burns off 400 additional calories, so you're burning a total of 1,900 calories a day. Your appetite does increase—but probably not by much, says Dr. Kenney. It might grow by 200 calories, to about 1,800 calories of food consumed daily. Compared with 1,900 calories burned, that makes for a negative calorie balance of 100 calories a day, which leads to weight loss. So exercise away—it really can balance the appetite to a healthy level.

9. Ask Yourself Why ▶ Before you eat, ask yourself why you want to eat. It may help you realize that it has nothing to do with hunger.

For most people, emotions are a major reason for overeating. "Eighty-five percent of my patients have psychological reasons for overeating," says Dr. Simonson. "And one of the major reasons is stress.

Stress makes you eat more quickly than anything else.

"Some people who are stressed out go for soft, creamy, comfort foods, like mashed potatoes with plenty of butter. Or they want baked foods, like a milk-and-cookies snack: It's the 'nothing-says-loving-like-something-from-the-oven' syndrome."

If you are turning to food in response to bad feelings, it's important to develop a strategy to feel better, says Dr. Simonson. "Before you eat, ask yourself, 'How am I feeling about myself right now? What's happened this week to upset me? Am I eating this because I'm hungry or because I'm upset?' "

Antistress measures, from counseling to yoga, can help you feel better and eat less. Above all, says Dr. Simonson, don't start a weight-loss program during a time of severe stress. "Always work on your emotional problems before you change your diet."

10. Know Your Own Triggers ▶ The sound and smell of sizzling sausage. The crunchy texture of popcorn. The smell, sight, sound and even texture of foods are the most powerful triggers we have to eat—and to overeat.

"I recently had a craving for a kosher hot dog," Dr. Simonson recalls, "not because I was hungry, but because I was thinking about the tight skin and how it goes 'pop' when you bite into it." Sometimes we eat things because they look good, even when they aren't. "Haven't we all eaten mediocre cookies, just because they looked delicious?" she asks.

And sometimes we eat them just because they're around. So eliminate the temptation by banishing fattening foods from the house. "Our eating is so dependent on external cues that just seeing foods makes us want to eat," says Dr. Simonson. If someone else in the family has to have sweets or high-fat foods, ask him to hide them somewhere where you can't find them.

Dr. Simonson's team has even found that slow, soft music makes people eat more slowly, take smaller bites and even enjoy the food more. It tastes better, says Dr. Simonson, because when you eat slowly you really smell

35

(continued on page 38)

AVOIDING APPETITE TURN-ONS

Want to gain a lot of weight in the unhealthiest way possible? Of course not. Yet millions of Americans regularly do the very things that turn their appetites on full throttle. Here are three big don'ts.

Don't diet or skip meals. Few things can increase your appetite like a prolonged restrictive diet, says Maria Simonson, Ph.D, Sc.D., director of the Health, Weight and Stress Clinic at Johns Hopkins Medical Institutions in Baltimore.

Psychologically, we overeat after starving "because we feel like we've been punishing ourselves. We want a reward," says Dr. Simonson. Physiologically, our body is doing what it can to fight starvation. It knows it's low on fuel, so our appetite eventually shoots up.

Even skipping meals can lead to a ravenous appetite, notes Wayne Callaway, M.D., obesity specialist and clinical professor at George Washington University in Washington, D.C. "People who skip breakfast or lunch tend to binge after dinner in the evening, instead of eating moderately. It's a common problem among chronic dieters."

The problem with skipping meals is that the blood sugar and glycogen that the body uses as fuel drop very low, signaling the body to demand more food and making you hungry.

Most responsible weight-loss experts these days are recommending that people worry less about cutting calories and focus instead on eating low-fat, high-carbohydrate, high-fiber foods. Those foods are less likely to be stored as fat, and they tend to reduce appetite and increase metabolic rate after meals so the body naturally limits the amount it takes in.

Don't hang out with the gang of two. "Fats and sweets are a deadly combination," says Thomas Wadden, Ph.D., director of the Center for Health Behavior at Syracuse University in New York. Each, by itself, heightens appetite. But the combination is by far the best way to shift the appetite into overdrive.

"Eating sweets can lead to a big increase in the amount

of sugar in the blood," explains Nori Geary, Ph.D., associate research professor at the Cornell University Medical Center in White Plains, New York. "That causes insulin levels to soar. Insulin stimulates the metabolism of sugars—not just the sugar you ate, but all sugars in the blood that the brain uses for fuel. In some people, the result is a lower blood sugar level than they started with. And that can turn up the appetite."

When fat is combined with carbohydrate, insulin levels are pushed up much more than with carbohydrate alone, says Dr. Kenney. And the combination pushes insulin far above what either of them can do alone, he notes.

"That's why it's better to avoid high-fat, high-sugar foods entirely. Very few people can get away with 'just a bite,' " Dr. Kenney says. If you do have an overwhelming sweet craving, go for a hard candy or a mint. "You just can't eat that many hard candies," says Dr. Kenney.

Don't count on swimming. Many scientists have searched for reasons to explain why swimming, an excellent cardiovascular and muscle workout, doesn't seem to trim off body fat as effectively as walking or other exercises. Dr. Kenney thinks it has to do with the fact that swimming, unlike other forms of exercise, does not raise the core body temperature. "And if it doesn't warm you up, it doesn't slim you down.

"Swimmers stay cool when they swim because the high heat capacity of water compared with air drains heat from the body," says Dr. Kenney. "So afterward, they're hungry not only from glycogen depletion but also because their bodies don't heat up. That may be why people tend to climb out of the pool ravenous but finish a fast walk hot, but not hungry." Most research suggests that swimmers, unlike walkers, runners and bicyclists, do not lose weight spontaneously.

This doesn't mean you should stop swimming, but it's important to be aware of the possibility of increased appetite and to counter it by being extra careful to eat only low-fat, high-fiber foods. And to lose weight, combine swimming with other exercises, such as walking or cycling.

the food—and odor enhances flavor.

Keeping a food record can help you identify these kinds of cues. For a couple of days, write down everything you eat and try to recall what made you start thinking about food—whether it was an advertisement or an emotion or an aroma. That helps you outthink a craving next time it happens.

6   Banish Belly Fat

Simple steps to a slimmer you.

Do you have a potbelly that makes you simmer? Did it sneak up on you over the years, bit by bit? Has it persisted despite round after round of gut-busting sit-ups? Despite deprivation diets that caused it to recede, then swell to an even greater size? Don't despair. That midriff mound may not be as immovable as you think.

This is good news, and not only for appearance' sake. There's something about belly fat in particular that raises the risk of heart disease, high blood pressure and diabetes, studies show. It seems to contribute to higher cholesterol levels as well. And in women, carrying your fat in front may raise the risk of both breast and endometrial cancer.

Specifically, researchers believe it's the fat that accumulates inside the abdominal cavity (visceral or depot fat), not the smaller layer of fat just below the skin (subcutaneous fat), that's to blame. How it raises the risk of these diseases, though, is not understood.

Why some people are more prone to develop a potbelly is also a bit of a mystery. The tendency is more common in men. Women who have the problem are often said to have an "apple" shape versus a "pear" shape, where more fat resides on the hips and thighs. But individuals of both sexes tend to expand at the waist as they age, research shows.

And while genetics and hormones do appear to play

a role, there is evidence that everyday behaviors are also to blame for bulging bellies.

The good news is that removing your "spare tire" will probably deflate the risks to your health—and give you a slimmer profile to boot!

Here's a seven-point potbelly-burning plan.

1. Go Easy on the Sauce ▶ If you're aiming to reduce a potbelly, first you've got to stop adding to it. And if you like to imbibe, cutting your alcohol intake may be key.

There really is such a thing as a beer belly, it seems. In a study of 1,628 men and women, those who quaffed more than two drinks a day had the largest waist-to-hip ratio (WHR), which is how doctors quantify potbellies. The drinkers had roughly twice as many large ratios among them as did the nondrinkers.

2. Stop Puffing ▶ In the same study, researchers at Stanford University School of Medicine and the University of California, San Diego, detected a similar effect for smoking. There were twice as many fat abdomens among those who lit up as among nonsmokers. Several other studies point the finger at smoking, too.

Some people continue to smoke because they're more worried about looking fat (some quitters gain a few pounds) than they are about the health hazards of smoking. If you keep smoking, you might weigh a bit less, but your weight may not be distributed in an attractive or healthy way.

3. Start Huffing ▶ The Stanford/University of California study found that lack of exercise was associated with inflating a spare tire in men.

And getting your mountain moving may help it disappear, other research shows. In a study at the University of Washington, when 15 older men (average age about 68) followed an endurance exercise training program for six months, they lost fat preferentially from their abdomen.

And though these men walked, jogged and biked for 45 to 60 minutes, five days a week, strenuous exercise

39

may not be necessary to bring about this result. It's possible that mild aerobic exercise over a long period will produce the same results or do even more.

One expert who believes that's true is Bryant Stamford, Ph.D., professor of allied health and director of health promotion at the University of Louisville in Kentucky. To burn off a belly, he says, exercise must do two things. First, it must start out vigorously enough to trigger a substantial adrenaline release.

"One of the jobs of adrenaline is to increase the free fatty acids in the bloodstream so the body can use them as fuel for activity," says Dr. Stamford. "And a prime location for that to occur is the stores of fat in the abdominal area." It may be that those fat cells are just particularly sensitive to adrenaline. In any case, you can probably get this effect from brisk walking, he says.

But the vigorous activities that mobilize this fat-for-fuel must then be followed by prolonged aerobic activities that will burn up the liberated fat. Walking at a comfortable pace fits the bill. "Just step up the pace or even jog a bit now and then to boost adrenaline output," says Dr. Stamford.

But you're not limited to walking. If you're gardening, for example, you might start out with some digging, a very vigorous activity. Then follow up with some raking or other sustained aerobic activity. "It's the combination that's probably going to be most helpful," says Dr. Stamford.

Just remember, in order to banish a belly, the foremost emphasis is on *aerobic*. Strength training doesn't directly burn fat as fuel. Over the long term, though, it can contribute mightily by building more muscle mass. Muscle burns more calories even at rest and can therefore help keep you from regaining lost fat.

4. Stop Throwing Fat at the Problem ▶ You've probably heard it before: The fat you eat is the fat you wear. And if you're someone who's prone to wearing it on your abdomen, reducing your fat intake is likely to be a good belly-busting strategy.

In a study of 124 women who each lost 10 to 15

pounds by cutting dietary fat and calories, 64 percent lost fat preferentially from their abdomen. Abdominal fat is actually easier to get rid of than fat carried like saddlebags, says David Schapira, M.D., chief of cancer prevention at the H. Lee Moffitt Cancer Center and Research Institute and professor of medicine at the University of South Florida College of Medicine in Tampa. "The fat cells on the abdomen are larger and less numerous than the ones on the buttocks and thighs. When you lose weight, you don't lose fat cells, they just shrink. And the ones that have the most potential for size reduction are the larger ones on the abdomen."

In most cases diet alone won't do the job on a monster midsection. Best bet: Use it as part of a comprehensive plan that includes exercise.

5. Don't Sweeten the Pot ▶ Fat may not be the only culprit in storing belly blubber, however. A dietary duet born in the USA may contribute heavily, according to Dr. Stamford. "It's typically American. We like to combine simple sugars and fats in the same meal—a hamburger, French fries and a cola, for example."

When the body gets a jolt of simple sugars, as from a soda, it releases lots of insulin in response. "Insulin is a storage-prone hormone," says Dr. Stamford. "It 'opens up' the fat cells, making them ready to store fat. Then here comes the fat from the burgers and fries, and bingo—the arrow is pointing toward storage."

The idea is controversial, but Dr. Stamford believes that people who tend to store more fat on their abdomen (called android or male-pattern obesity) may suffer in particular from this kind of meal because the abdominal fat cells are very active. "They can lose fat quickly but also can suck up fat quickly from the bloodstream," he says.

"To get rid of fat, you've got to stop the flow. Go on a low-fat diet, and when you do consume fat, don't consume simple sugars with it. Then you won't be replenishing abdominal fat, and you're going to point the arrow the other way and begin to draw it out. And that's when exercise is going to be extremely helpful."

6. Lose It Once ▶ Weight's more dangerous the second time around, it seems. Researchers at Yale University and the University of California, Davis, found a significant association between a higher WHR and a higher degree of weight cycling—losing and regaining weight repeatedly. "Animal studies support this observation," says Patricia Johnson, Ph.D., professor of nutrition and animal physiology at the University of California, Davis.

Researchers aren't sure why weight cycling puts more fat on the abdomen. One leading theory is that this kind of yo-yo dieting increases fat consumption. In one study, for example, lab animals that were made to lose weight and then allowed to regain selected a higher-fat diet than animals that had never lost weight.

In another study, women who had regained lost weight ate more candy and chocolate than women who either maintained weight loss or had no history of weight loss and regain. "There does seem to be evidence for a shift in fat preference as a result of cycling behavior," says Dr. Johnson.

Top obesity researcher Kelly Brownell, Ph.D., of the Yale University Department of Psychology, recommends the following measures to avoid weight cycling.

■ Before beginning a weight-loss program, make sure you're extremely motivated.

■ Also, make sure you're committed to maintaining a healthy diet and increased exercise for life.

■ And don't start a weight-loss program under difficult life circumstances that you feel may jeopardize your chances for success.

■ Stick with a sensible diet that relies on fruit, vegetables and other low-fat fare, and emphasize slow, gradual weight loss.

42

7. Take a Firm Stand ▶ While a lot of gut-busting sit-ups may give you very finely toned abdominal muscles, nobody will ever see them if they're covered with a layer of fat, says Doug Semenick, director of the Wellness Program and strength coach at the University of Louisville. And your belly bulge won't budge if a large pot of intra-abdominal fat is pushing your middle out. However, once the fat is whittled away by diet and aerobic exercise, "various abdominal exercises can make the area firmer, and it may appear smaller under your clothes," says Semenick.

Just remember: While abdominal exercises may help to improve your shape a bit, they're not going to bring the health benefits of actually removing belly fat.

To firm tummy muscles, Dr. Stamford recommends starting with isometric squeezes. To do them, tense your abdominal muscles to the maximum and hold for six to ten seconds. Relax, then repeat several times.

Later you can move on to the bent-knee, half sit-ups known as crunches or abdominal curls: Lie on your back with your knees bent. Cross your arms on your chest. Lift your head up toward your chest. Keep going until you lift your shoulder blades slightly off the ground. Hold for two seconds, then lie back down.

Alternate this curl with ones in which you curl up toward your left knee and then toward your right knee so you work the obliques (muscles on the sides of the abdomen). For example, curl up to the left, then down, then to the middle, then down, then to the right. Repeat for a set of 10 (30 crunches in all). Once you can do a set of 10, you can add a couple of repetitions or another set.

"I find in my testing here at Louisville that roughly 80 to 90 percent of the women have some weakness of their lower abdominal muscles in particular," says Semenick. "Especially following childbirth, those muscles can be lax and loose. And that can contribute to looking like you have a paunch down there."

Medical Breakthroughs

Healing Lights 7

Exciting new therapies
that can brighten your life.

Meet the fictional Franklin family of the not-too-distant future: Evelyn Franklin, a senior executive, often jets back and forth from New York to Paris. To keep jet lag from dragging her down, she uses a portable light-therapy box that the airline offers in-flight.

Her husband, Tom, mans a military defense post—on a shift starting at midnight. He uses artificial light to make night mimic day, so his wits are razor-sharp in the predawn hours.

Their son, Tim, is honor-roll material, except in winter, when he can barely get out of bed to attend classes, due to lethargy and drowsiness that accompany his seasonal depression. So as he sleeps, a computer-controlled light box nearby simulates an early sunrise, making it a breeze to get out and tackle calculus on a cold, dark day. He awakes refreshed, alert and upbeat.

This future scenario is fast becoming our present. In fact, sizzling new medical therapies incorporating light are being used for a wide range of disorders, including such hard-to-treat conditions such as psoriasis, midwinter depression and menstrual irregularity.

Seasonal Affective Disorder

For a small percentage of the adult population, it happens every winter: insomnia, lethargy, depression and a craving for sweets. Then once winter fades and the sun reappears, these symptoms vanish. This phenomenon is called seasonal affective disorder (SAD).

The shorter winter days ration our sunlight, which our body's clock needs to keep our sleep/wake cycles regulated. For most people, this rationing isn't a problem. But according to circadian rhythm researchers, in some people the light shortage throws the cycle off, which may bring on the dark mood.

(continued on page 48)

HOW TO GET AN EYEFUL

If you think you might have seasonal affective disorder (SAD), your first step should be to see your physician. He or she can help you get the bright-light therapy you need. In this kind of therapy, light must get to the brain through the eyes. Here are the options.

Try simple steps. "If a patient's habits or finances make a light box an unrealistic choice, I have him take a walk or do some gardening," says Daniel F. Kripke, M.D., a professor of psychiatry at the University of California, San Diego. "Of course, I wouldn't say that to folks in Fairbanks, Alaska. Some patients in warm locations will walk, while others in colder climates may try light boxes."

One study actually had SAD patients take morning walks and found that those who received a minimal daily exposure of one hour of sunlight got some benefit in their treatment of SAD.

Wearing a sunscreen is mandatory, of course, even in SAD therapy. After all, the light has to get to your eyes, not your skin.

Camp by a lamp. Some people stuck in dark places may feel better with simple exposure to normal room light. Research, however, suggests that people with SAD may need higher intensities of light (light boxes described below offer roughly five to ten times the light of an ordinary lamp).

"Try a regular indoor light or a vigorous walk first—before you start spending money," says Michael Terman, Ph.D., director of the Winter Depression Program at the New York Psychiatric Institute.

Light boxes are what's used in the majority of SAD studies. They're about two feet by two feet and angled toward the person's face so that the screen is about 18 inches from the eyes. They can give off up to 10,000 lux (light is measured in luxes, with normal indoor light being 500 lux). About 2,500 lux—the lower end of power used in some treatments—equals the level at 15 minutes after sunrise. About 10,000 lux—the high end of treatment—is equal to about 40 minutes after sunrise. With light treatment, the relationship is dose-dependent—a half hour of 10,000 lux is as effective as two hours at 2,500 lux.

Most studies find that early-morning sessions ranging from 30 minutes to two hours using varying intensities of light can bring on improvements within a week.

The light source is usually white fluorescent and doesn't require UV light for therapeutic effect. The boxes cost $300 to $550.

During treatment, you sit at a table with the light box nearby. You don't look into it—you simply keep your head and eyes toward the light, concentrating on a meal or book illuminated by the lights.

Symptoms can return if treatment stops. Most users need to maintain a consistent daily schedule, beginning in the fall or winter and usually continuing until spring, when the sun starts hanging around more.

Side effects are minor—including eye irritation and redness. The most dramatic side effect is a kind of overactive state, a restless high. Light boxes are available over the counter, but haven't received approval by the Food and Drug Administration.

Get up for an artificial sunrise. Some researchers are now testing a twilight simulator, a device that resembles a computer and mimics a sunrise. It shines light of gradually increasing intensity toward the eyes of the sleeper, stimulating the eyes through the eyelids at a time when they are supposedly sensitive to light.

One small study had a group of SAD patients compare the artificial dawn to a basic alarm clock. With the fake dawn, six of the eight subjects reported full remissions of their SAD symptoms, though the benefits wore off once they went back to the clock.

That's not the only mechanism behind the malaise, however. Winter's light thievery may also toy with chemicals in the brain that instigate depression and cravings for sweets. One theory points to melatonin, a hormone secreted by the pineal gland, a walnut-size structure behind the midbrain. Research suggests that the more melatonin there is, the more likely you'll feel drowsy or depressed. And since melatonin production peaks in darkness—while sunlight suppresses it—winter's light shortage may trigger a chemical cascade of unhappiness.

"Evidence also points to another brain chemical, serotonin, which decreases in dark, cold times—suggesting that our craving for carbohydrates is our attempt to restore serotonin function," says Norman E. Rosenthal, M.D., chief of the Outpatient Studies Clinical Psychobiology Branch at the National Institute of Mental Health in Bethesda, Maryland.

SAD prevalence increases with geographical latitude. (In Florida, less than 2 percent of the population might have it, compared with 10 percent in New Hampshire.) The farther north the location, the shorter the average winter day and the higher the rates of SAD.

"Studies are repeatedly showing, however, that bright-light therapy can offer consistent, quick relief to people suffering from SAD," says Michael Terman, Ph.D., director of the Winter Depression Program at the New York Psychiatric Institute and Columbia Presbyterian Medical Center in New York City.

In a review of several studies, researchers found that response rates to light treatment (response being a significant drop in symptoms) averaged 60 percent, compared with 20 percent for dim-light placebos. Although studies of long-term treatment results are lacking, evidence suggests that benefits may last throughout the winter if the treatment is kept up.

Often, light treatment is used to bolster the power of antidepressant medication. "Some patients receive just a partial benefit from drugs alone," says Dr. Terman. "Once light is added, the full response may kick in." Photosensitive drugs—which make your skin more sensitive to light—shouldn't be used along with light treatment, however.

Delayed Sleep-Phase Syndrome

If you can't fall asleep until the wee hours of the morning (2:30 or 3 A.M.) and then can't wake up in time for a normal workday, bright light may be the answer.

"People who have had delayed sleep-phase syndrome for years have seen it disappear for the first time in their lives using light therapy," says Dr. Terman. If you get a dose of bright light in the morning, your day may start earlier so you fall asleep at a decent time that night. And for someone with a natural tendency to conk out right after dinner but wake up in the early-morning hours, bright light at night may work to delay bedtime, too. (As a rule, light around dawn resets the body clock to an earlier hour, while evening light resets it to a later hour.)

In one study, bright light was used on 20 patients who on average couldn't get to sleep until 1 A.M. at least four times a week for as long as three years. Two hours of morning exposure to bright light, plus light restriction at night, successfully altered the troubled sleepers' circadian rhythms. When they received a placebo treatment of only a low-powered light, there was no change in their circadian rhythms. Sleep and morning alertness improved significantly during the active treatment.

In another study, light was used on a group of 25 chronic oversleepers. These folks commonly sleep right through their clanging alarm clocks and then feel drowsy for one to three hours after getting up. A low-intensity 150-watt floodlight was placed six feet from the sleepers' heads. It was timed to turn on ten minutes before the alarm went off and an hour before their normal wake-up time. Sleepers were to get up and turn off the light—but not return to bed. Fifteen patients reported full responses—with at least two successive weeks of getting up successfully with the light and being fully alert. Nine patients had partial responses (in which improvement wasn't consistent). One patient had no response. The mechanism isn't known, but because human eyelids are translucent, it could be that light affects the central nervous system during sleep.

49

Jet Lag

If you're a traveler who frequently flies across several time zones, jet lag is baggage you wouldn't mind losing. The lag's not due only to long flights in small seats that keep you cramped, irritable and awake for hours. It also results from the time required to synchronize the body's circadian rhythms to the night-and-day cycle of the new environment.

"You can actually measure the effects of jet lag for up to a few weeks, even after your sleep/wake schedule returns to normal," says Dr. Terman. That's where harnessing light may help—by fooling your body clock into a new time zone. "It might not be too far off in the future when you'll be able to get on a plane, whip out a portable light box and prepare for your destination," he says.

When you arrive in Paris from New York without any light preparation, for example, your body still thinks it's in the Big Apple, where it's midnight and time for bed. In an hour or two, though, the Parisians will be up, croissant and café au lait in hand, ready to do business. "It hasn't been proven yet, but by using bright-light treatment to advance your rhythms before leaving the East Coast, you may be able to put yourself in sync with the local population in Paris," says Dr. Terman. In this case, you'd probably need to get up earlier the day before and use lights (or a walk in the bright sun) to kick your body clock into advance gear.

You can also get some sunny support upon arrival, provided it's a clear-sky afternoon. Studies suggest that travelers adapt faster to a time-zone shift if they stay outdoors on arrival rather than lounge in their hotel rooms.

Night-Shift Work

For over seven million Americans, their work schedule demands activity at night and sleep during the day—a routine that flies in the face of the body's natural night/day circadian rhythms. "Here, out-of-sync circadian phases could lead to serious harm due to fatigue-related accidents," says Dr. Terman.

Research using bright light on night-shift workers

suggests, however, that cognitive performance at hours that normally show a terrible slump—4:30 to 5:30 A.M.— may be enhanced. In an analysis of ten studies involving night-shift workers, researchers found that the circadian rhythms of workers could be successfully shifted after bright-light exposure at night and complete darkness during the day for four days. These shifts resulted in a significant boost in both alertness and cognitive performance during the work hours. Plus, the workers slept two hours longer during the day. The workers who didn't undergo bright-light therapy saw no such improvement.

"This is a new field, but I'm confident that light therapy will offer real benefits to people in this kind of work," says Dr. Terman.

Midwinter Insomnia

Imagine spending two months straight with no natural daylight. Outside, it's totally dark—with only a few hours of dim light per day. That's what the folks in Tromso, Norway, endure from November 20 to January 20 each year. During this time many people experience what's called midwinter insomnia—a difficulty falling asleep that lasts throughout the dark period.

Some light-treatment research has been devoted to this problem, with modest but encouraging results. In one such study, a group of Tromsonians used bright light early in the morning. They were able to feel drowsy earlier than usual in the evening—possibly due to shifting their biological clocks. Their results were better than those of the comparison group receiving no treatment, although the treatment's effectiveness didn't match the estimated effectiveness of sleeping medications.

Nonseasonal Depression

Only a few studies have tried to determine whether the treatment can help people with nonseasonal depression—and the results, so far, have been mixed. Two preliminary studies using only a single dose of bright light found significant, though small, improvements in depression ratings among the patients. In another study, seven nonseasonal depressives experienced a 13 percent reduction in their ratings of depression.

Irregular Menstrual Cycles

Researchers two decades ago reported that a 100-watt bedside light might shorten and regulate menstrual cycles among women with long and irregular ones. "More recently we repeated this experiment and got the same results," says Daniel F. Kripke, M.D., a professor of psychiatry at the University of California, San Diego.

In his research, seven volunteers slept with the same-power bulb by their bedside from days 13 to 17 of their cycle, while a control group used a dim red bulb. The women getting the 100-watt light experienced cycles shortened from an average of 45.7 days to roughly 33 days, while also having less cycle irregularity. "This needs more research, but it offers intriguing implications for treating infertility and improving upon contraception," says Dr. Kripke.

Bulimia

People with bulimia often show signs of winter depression, with symptoms of their eating disorder getting worse during that time, too. (Bulimia is characterized by eating lots of food in a short time span, followed by purging.) That's why some researchers speculated that light therapy might work here, too. One study targeted 17 bulimic patients—with roughly half of them experiencing a seasonal variety that worsens during winter.

For two weeks the group received the therapy using bright light, then they were switched to two weeks of dim lighting. Patients weren't told which was the active treatment. "During the bright-light therapy the subjects experienced a 50 percent reduction in the number of binges and purges, as well as in their feelings of depression," says Raymond W. Lam, M.D., assistant professor of psychiatry at the University of British Columbia, Vancouver. In the control group, the bulimia lessened about 20 percent.

As mentioned earlier, it's possible that bright light may help reset the inner clock disturbed by winter's diminishing sunlight, while also correcting disturbances involving the chemical serotonin. "That chemical is involved in appetite regulation as well as mood regulation," says Dr. Lam.

Right now, however, it's far from clear whether this treatment is truly effective for bulimia. This was a small, preliminary study, and much larger studies are needed. Anyone who feels they may have an eating disorder should see their doctor before trying any experimental treatment.

Vitiligo

When an ancient Egyptian had this disorder—characterized by white patches on the skin—he'd usually have a spot of tea and a nap on the beach. The therapy hasn't changed much since then. That's because he was simply using a primitive version of a proven therapy called PUVA (psoralens and ultraviolet A, or psoralen, chemotherapy).

"People would remove a substance called psoralen from various plants, eat it or make tea with it, and then expose themselves to the sun," says Warwick L. Morison, M.D., associate professor of dermatology and research at the National Cancer Institute at Johns Hopkins Hospital in Baltimore. "And they'd get better."

These psoralen compounds, usually harmless by themselves, are found not just in plant seeds but also in fruits and vegetables (limes, lemons, celery, parsley and lettuce, for example). They have the capacity to interact with light, producing a chemical reaction that transforms the substance into a natural pesticide. "An insect would fly along, eat the seeds, become sensitive to the sun and get cooked," says Dr. Morison.

"Some clever person picked up on this and applied it to vitiligo, and that's how we got the idea for PUVA therapy," he says. It's been tested and is now a proven therapy.

In contemporary treatment, oral or topical psoralens are given to the patient. Two to four hours later he or she is exposed to full-body UV light. "The treatment here works by stimulating the pigment-producing cells in the hair follicles so they'll come out and reach the skin," says Dr. Morison. The therapy might call for 150 to 200 treatments given over one to two years—breaking down to about 1½ doses of PUVA per week. "If you combine PUVA with thin skin grafts, however, you can cut the therapy down to 50 treatments," he says.

Psoriasis

The chronic skin disease psoriasis leaves its calling card as itchy, white, scaly patches. The disease occurs when skin cells start dividing when they shouldn't—a devastating and often unstoppable process. "Ultraviolet light stops the skin cells from dividing, resulting in very dramatic cures in many cases," says Meyrick Peak, M.D., senior scientist with the Biological and Medical Research Division of the Department of Chemistry at the University of Georgia in Athens. "Although there may be an elevated long-term risk for developing some skin tumors from this treatment, psoriasis can be disfiguring and painful enough to call for this treatment," he says. Premature aging and freckling may also occur.

"As long as UV is used in a controlled fashion, the side effects can be minimized," says Dr. Morison. If the disease is limited to just the hands and feet, for example, then special equipment will target those areas only. If it's all over the body, the person would enter what looks like a horizontal phone booth with light bulbs all around. "Despite the side effects, in many cases UV treatment may be the safest and most effective treatment," says Dr. Morison.

In fact, in study settings, 88 to 90 percent of patients with psoriasis who are treated with PUVA respond favorably. "The treatment usually involves 30 PUVA sessions spanning ten weeks," says Dr. Morison. "When the disease is controlled, maintenance therapy might involve one treatment per week or one every two weeks," he says. Flare-ups after the initial therapy occur in roughly 20 percent of all patients.

Jaundice

Characterized by yellow pigmentation of the skin, jaundice is usually brought on by hyperbilirubinemia, or excessive blood concentrations of a bile pigment called bilirubin. It affects roughly 5 percent of all infants born each year.

"We've found that the blue light of the spectrum is most effective in treating this problem," says Dr. Morison. Blue light somehow changes the bilirubin so it's able to exit the blood more easily. The treatment's widely used because it is innocuous—doing away with more intensive treatments like perfusions, where blood is passed through a pig liver or some other medium. The therapy is straightforward: The baby is placed under a bank of blue lights and remains there until the light does the trick and the skin turns its normal color, which takes a few hours.

Skin Cancer

"The very thing that can lead to skin cancer may also cure it," says Dr. Peak. In photodynamic therapy, dyes that absorb light are injected into tumors, and then the cancers are exposed to light. "The light's photons are absorbed by the pigment held by the dye, which becomes chemically reactive—causing the cancer cells to die," says Dr. Peak.

Still considered experimental in this country, this therapy has been used in China for over 20 years and has been very good at getting rid of surface tumors. "I've seen tremendous before-and-after pictures of people who once had large facial tumors and then posttreatment looking perfectly normal," says Dr. Peak.

"It's currently being tested here for basal and squamous cell cancers," says Nicholas J. Lowe, M.D., clinical professor of dermatology at the University of Southern California, Los Angeles, School of Medicine and the Southern California Dermatology and Psoriasis Center in Santa Monica. "The concern with it, however, is unwanted phototoxicity—anyone under treatment is likely to be sensitive to sunlight for long periods of time."

Light has also been harnessed in other ways to fight skin cancers. Extracorporeal photochemotherapy (also called photopheresis), an experimental treatment, involves removing white cells from the blood and passing them through a machine that exposes them to UVA light. The patient has already taken a psoralen drug— making this an out-of-body form of PUVA. The cells containing psoralen pass through, get zapped by light and then are put back into the person.

"In the case of a skin lymphoma called mycosis fungoides, the condition seems to improve after three or four treatments," says Dr. Morison. (Lymphocytes are white blood cells usually found in our blood. But a family of them live in the skin and can become cancerous.)

"Photopheresis can be effective, but for only a select group of patients with severe lymphoma that involves much of the body," says Dr. Lowe. "For disease in the early stages, PUVA therapy is likely to be a better choice for treatment."

Bladder Cancer

Current research is also testing light in the treatment of bladder tumors. In a preliminary study out of the Netherlands, phototherapy was used to treat bladder cancer in 12 patients. After three months, all patients were free of detectable disease, but recurrences did occur in three of them. In this experimental treatment, physicians were able to control the uniformity of the light dose and measure continuously the total dose at the bladder wall during treatment—considered an advancement in the therapy.

"If you put a laser into the bladder and shine a bright light at the cancer cells containing a dye, you might clear the bladder of the cancers," says Dr. Peak. "You might also flood an operation site with a dye or drug, shine a light before sewing the patient up, and kill any cells that might escape."

Lupus

Systemic lupus erythematosus, an autoimmune disease, wreaks havoc on the skin, kidneys, blood vessels, nervous system, heart and other internal organs. Women get it about nine or ten times more often than men. Steroids—used to combat the illness—are unfortunately often saddled with serious side effects. Now researchers are turning to light as a potential therapy to ease the dependence on drugs.

In one study involving 15 patients, those who received light therapy with UVA-1 (a type of UVA) had significantly reduced symptoms of the disease compared with those who were treated with a placebo. The light was applied in a device much like a tanning bed two to five times a week for 18 weeks. UVA-1 light has almost no side effects, unlike UVB light, which is toxic to lupus patients.

"The patients had decreases in joint pain, headaches, sleeplessness and need for medication," says Hugh McGrath, M.D., associate professor of medicine at the Section of Rheumatology at the Louisiana State University Medical Center in Shreveport. "The chief benefit was a decline in fatigue, which patients really notice and where drugs aren't as helpful." But since lupus symptoms can come and go on their own, and because this was a small study, more research is needed to figure out if light is really as effective against lupus as it appears.

8 Get the Jump on Joint Pain

*Powerful treatments help
keep arthritis under control.*

You have a pain in your hip that comes and goes, and you've noticed stiffness in your shoulder. "Just a part of growing older," you think. "Not much use in going to the doctor—not much anyone can do."

Today that couldn't be less true. "Pain is not something that should be there merely because you're getting older," says Kenneth D. Brandt, M.D., professor of medicine and head of the Rheumatology Division at the Indiana University School of Medicine in Indianapolis. "It's not part of normal aging."

Doctors are now emphasizing not only that in many cases early treatment of arthritis can minimize the damage but also that now there are different, more effective treatments available. The medication or treatment your doctor prescribes today for arthritis is likely to be very different from what she would have prescribed five years ago—and researchers are hard at work testing even more advanced forms of treatment.

"There's literally an explosion of information in arthritis research," says David S. Pisetsky, M.D., Ph.D., co-director of the Duke University Arthritis Center, professor of medicine in the Department of Rheumatology at Duke University Medical Center in Durham, North Carolina, and author of *The Duke University Medical Center Book of Arthritis.* "The approach to many arthritis problems is changing every year," he says.

No Time to Be Stoic

Something that's news to many people—including the six million Americans who believe they have arthritis but have never seen a doctor for treatment—is the importance of seeing a doctor when you first start experiencing joint pain or swelling.

A doctor and only a doctor can tell you what type of arthritis you have—or if your joint pain is caused by another problem. This is important because treatments for the two most common types of arthritis—osteoarthritis (OA) and rheumatoid arthritis (RA)—are very different.

RA involves severe inflammation that can seriously damage your joints and lead to other complications, and doctors now believe that beginning treatment early is crucial to help avoid or delay irreversible joint damage that occurs in the first few years of the disease. In OA, it's mostly cartilage and sometimes bone that breaks down. If it's untreated, you can lose mobility because of the pain and stiffness as the cartilage that lines and cushions your joints deteriorates.

"If you have joint problems, you need to see a doctor early and find out if this is RA or another form of arthritis," says Dr. Pisetsky. "If we begin treatment early, we may help the body restore balance earlier. What I don't like to see is patients delaying medical care to the point that the ability of the physician to intervene is diminished."

It isn't as crucial to see a doctor early with OA because the primary problem is cartilage breakdown, which can't yet be stopped. But early treatment can prevent joints from "freezing up" or losing mobility because pain has kept you from moving them.

"If you have pain in your joint because of arthritis, you have a tendency not to move it beyond the point of pain," says Arthur I. Grayzel, M.D., senior vice president for medical affairs for the Arthritis Foundation. "And you can lose the normal range of motion if you don't use the joint." That means you can't bend or straighten your joint as far as you used to be able to.

Finally, doctors today recommend a complete approach that includes physical therapy, an exercise program and differences in the way you move. "It's a team approach to arthritis," says Dr. Pisetsky. "Is your diet right? Have you had physical therapy? Are you in an exercise program? Are you protecting your joints?"

Because muscle weakness may affect how a joint functions, it's crucial to maintain muscle tone. "It's a good idea to use an exercise program established by a professional," says Dr. Grayzel. "The program should have several goals, including moving your joints through their complete range of motion so you don't lose mobility."

And exercise can make a dramatic difference: A study of 102 people with OA of the knee found that after eight weeks, the people who participated in a supervised walking program had less pain, used less medication and were more mobile than the nonwalking group.

Rheumatoid Arthritis: Overturning Conventional Treatment

In rheumatoid arthritis, treatment has been turned upside down. For much of the last quarter-century, treatment of RA has followed a conventional "pyramid" approach that began with routine treatment that included physical therapy, salicylates (like aspirin) and anti-inflammatory drugs called NSAIDs (nonsteroidal anti-inflammatory drugs). Only as the disease progressed did doctors move up the pyramid to more aggressive treatments such as prednisone, gold, penicillamine and methotrexate.

The rationale behind this treatment was that RA was a relatively benign disease and that the possible risks or side effects of the more aggressive treatments weren't worth it, says Kenneth R. Wilske, M.D., head of clinical rheumatology and clinical immunology at Virginia Mason Clinic and clinical professor of medicine at the University of Washington in Seattle.

But this conventional treatment wasn't working for patients with aggressive RA, says Dr. Wilske. It might have relieved pain short-term, but it did little or nothing to stop the progression of the disease. "This aggressive disease is anything but benign," says Dr. Wilske. "Half of the people with RA may be incapacitated at the 5- to 6-year point, and 90 percent may be incapacitated after 20 years."

Researchers have shown that people with aggressive RA have long-term survival rates after ten years that approach those of people with some types of leukemia or advanced coronary artery disease. "This is an aggressive, life-threatening disease," says Dr. Wilske. "The length and quality of people's lives are impaired."

Because of this, and because studies show that 90 percent of joint damage occurs in the first few years of the disease, Dr. Wilske and other doctors recommend inverting that traditional pyramid for people with aggressive RA and starting treatment with the most effective drugs to stop or slow down damage before it occurs.

"There seems to be a brief, several-year window before the worst joint damage occurs," he says. "If you can inhibit that inflammatory reaction, then you have a much better chance of preventing joint damage." At that point, he says, the more potent, more toxic drugs can be dropped and treatment continued with safer drugs.

It's important to realize, however, that this aggressive treatment isn't warranted with all patients. Not only is a definite diagnosis of RA necessary, but additional factors must be considered to separate people with the more aggressive form of RA from those with the less destructive type—which doesn't warrant the use of the more toxic drugs.

"The best person to make this determination is a rheumatologist," says Dr. Wilske. "That's a doctor who specializes in diagnosing and treating arthritis."

Meet the Rheumatoid Arthritis Drugs ▶ These more aggressive agents include drugs called DMARDs (disease-modifying antirheumatic drugs) and immuno-suppressives (also called cytotoxic agents), all aimed at long-term control of inflammation. Initially physicians were reluctant to prescribe these drugs because of possible toxicity, and originally they were often prescribed in overly high doses, says Dr. Wilske.

Today these drugs are often used in combination and in lower doses or are given intermittently, both measures that can help reduce toxicity problems. "People are beginning to find that combination therapy may be no more or less toxic than the use of NSAIDs," says Dr. Wilske.

The DMARDs include oral or injected gold; chloro-quine or hydroxychloroquine, an antimalarial drug;

61

sulfasalazine, a combination of a sulfa drug and a salicylate; and penicillamine. The immunosuppressive drugs include methotrexate, azathioprine and cyclophosphamide. Corticosteroids such as prednisone are used by some to control inflammation until the DMARD takes effect.

"Nobody knows exactly how these drugs work," says Dr. Wilske. "But we do know how quickly they take effect. Cortisone starts working almost immediately, methotrexate works in one to two months and the others start to work within several months." There's no question that methotrexate is the star of these treatments, doctors agree, because of its rapid action and relative lack of side effects. Possible side effects from these drugs can include things such as rashes, liver damage and kidney and lung problems.

Treatments of the Future ▶ Most treatments for RA involve controlling the immune system, because experts suspect it's an immune response that causes the inflammation. This unfortunately has meant blocking beneficial immune responses as well. Ideally, medicines would block only the unwanted inflammation.

Researchers are investigating treatments that target cells that cause inflammation before it occurs. One approach is an antibody aimed at immune response cells called CD4 T cells, which researchers believe are the major cells causing the inflammation of RA. "It makes sense that if you reduce the function of those cells, you'd see improvement in RA," says Dr. Pisetsky. This is done by sending in monoclonal (specialized) antibodies targeted specifically to eliminate the CD4 T cells.

You don't want to wipe out all the cells, however, because they also help you fight infections such as flu and viruses. "What seems to happen is that you get at least a transient reduction in the number of CD4 T cells, and when they come back, a new level of immune function is established," explains Dr. Pisetsky.

Researchers at the University of Texas Southwestern Medical Center in Dallas are investigating another possibility: using specific antibodies targeted at cells'

ARTHRITIS: GETTING THE RIGHT MEDICAL CARE

If you wake up in the morning feeling a bit stiff and achy, it's okay to try a pain reliever such as aspirin or acetaminophen. But if you have persistent symptoms that last for two weeks or more, it's time to see a doctor.

Your family doctor is a good starting point. If you have osteoarthritis, your doctor can prescribe suitable treatment. Perhaps you need little more than over-the-counter medications for pain relief and range-of-motion exercises to keep the joint mobile. Even so, it's important to see your doctor to select the right medications and to help you make changes that may reduce joint damage.

A person with osteoarthritis needs a comprehensive program that includes exercises, ways of coping with pain, learning how to protect thejoints and perhaps some lifestyle changes. Once a program is set up, a patient can be taught how to adjust dosage according to symptoms.

If your family physician suspects that you may have rheumatoid arthritis or perhaps another problem, she should refer you to a specialist for evaluation. "Everyone with significant symptoms—like persistent joint swelling and tenderness, morning stiffness and fatigue—that suggest rheumatoid arthritis should see a rheumatologist," says David S. Pisetsky, M.D., Ph.D., co-director of the Duke University Arthritis Center and professor of medicine in the Department of Rheumatology at Duke University Medical Center in Durham, North Carolina. "This is an area of medicine that's changing rapidly. So you should avail yourself of someone who's on top of the latest developments in the field—that is, a rheumatologist."

Optimally, your family doctor and rheumatologist work together as a team; your doctor can monitor your progress on the treatment the specialist recommends.

63

adhesion molecules that act as "traffic cops" and direct immune cells to certain parts of the body. "The idea is to keep these cells from getting into the joint where they will cause arthritis," says researcher Arthur Kavanaugh, M.D., assistant professor of internal medicine. Preliminary test results in people with severe arthritis look promising, he says—although it's still a long road to developing a medication that's available to the public.

"These kinds of specific therapies are what most people believe is the future of arthritis treatment," says Dr. Kavanaugh.

Osteoarthritis:
Fitting the Dose to the Symptom

"Fifteen years ago I would lecture on osteoarthritis and people would fall asleep," says Roy Altman, M.D., professor of medicine at the University of Miami School of Medicine and chief of the Arthritis Section at the Miami Veterans Administration Medical Center. "Now they're staying awake." What's happening in this field? There's still no cure for OA, but treatment methods are changing and scientists are trying to develop new medications to halt the cartilage breakdown.

Reach for OTCs ▶ For many years doctors routinely prescribed NSAIDs for OA. In a study at the Indiana University School of Medicine, however, researchers found that patients responded just as well to over-the-counter pain relievers such as low-dose ibuprofen and acetaminophen as they did to a more potent—and more expensive—prescription-strength anti-inflammatory. The point is that not everyone needs an anti-inflammatory.

"There are many reasons why people with OA hurt," says Dr. Altman. "Sometimes it's inflammation, sometimes it's the bone around the joint, sometimes it's muscles in spasm." While prescription anti-inflammatory drugs may well relieve the pain, they not only cost more, they also have a higher risk for causing ulcers and other complications.

The preferred method today is treating the specific

symptom, says Dr. Brandt, coauthor of the Indiana University study. "For some patients, over-the-counter acetaminophen is not adequate, and they require NSAIDs," says Dr. Brandt. "On the other hand, there is a substantial number of patients for whom acetaminophen will suffice, especially when combined with other things such as physical therapy." Still others can eventually toss away all their pills, he says.

On the Horizon ▶ The medication you receive for OA today—whether prescription or over-the-counter—is aimed solely at relieving your pain and improving mobility. Scientists, however, are searching for a way to stop the cartilage breakdown that causes the damage.

Your cartilage is living tissue, and it has cells whose job is to produce new tissue and scavenge the old. In OA the scavenging process has gone awry, and more tissue is being picked up than being put down.

"There are probably 100 medications being tested now aimed at altering the process so the cartilage doesn't break down at all," says Dr. Altman. "I think how we treat OA will change dramatically in the next decade."

For more information, contact the Arthritis Foundation at P.O. Box 19000, Atlanta, GA 30326; (800) 283-7800.

9   The Well-Mannered Tummy

Dozens of tips for taming the tigers in your tank.

You've just wolfed down a salami sub and fries. Normally you wouldn't be caught dead in this grease pit, but in the rush to get out of the house this morning, you forgot your lunch. You have only a half hour before you have to return to a desk sagging under the weight of countless memos and reports, all of which must be cleared away by five o'clock, so you won't be late to pick up your daughter at day care. You've just returned to your desk when you are seized by the sudden, irresistible urge to stand up and run to the bathroom.

It's not funny, especially if your insides are in an uproar. Sometimes the villain is just a passing flu bug. Maybe it was something you ate or something that's just eating you. For whatever reason, your insides occasionally respond with uncomfortable, sometimes noisy, often embarrassing symptoms: hiccups, burps, heartburn, constipation, diarrhea and more.

So what do you do? For immediate action, try the following tips and recommendations from top gastrointestinal experts.

Belching

Most of the time, a belch or a burp (the forceful regurgitation of air from the stomach or esophagus) is a timely and helpful thing. But if you burp more than just after a meal—if, indeed, you belch frequently—you may be unconsciously swallowing air. Some people eat too fast, so they unconsciously swallow a lot of air. Some swallow air as they chew gum, suck hard candies or smoke. Quite a few people do it simply because they're nervous swallowers. And carbonated soft drinks are also well-known belch producers.

So the obvious thing to do is try to avoid those things, like chewing gum and smoking, that stimulate saliva (and swallowing). It may help to avoid drinking out of cans or bottles. If high-speed eating is a habit of yours, by all means slow down and chew completely. And those who swallow unconsciously, out of anxiety, often find that the belching stops once they become aware of the cause. Over-the-counter antacids, particularly those containing simethicone, may help break up those uncomfortable gas bubbles.

Hiccups

It all starts with spasmodic contractions of the diaphragm, a muscle that's located below the lungs and is used in breathing. The contractions close the glottis, the muscular flap that prevents food from going down your windpipe. When the glottis closes forcefully, the resulting noise is a hiccup. The nerves that control the muscles of breathing and respiration become irritated, prompting the diaphragm to do its version of the Mexican hat dance.

There are some age-old remedies that are said to help. Hiccups often can be alleviated by increasing the amount of carbon dioxide in your blood. You can do this by repeatedly holding your breath or breathing with a paper bag over your nose and mouth, says Carla Ginsburg, M.D., assistant professor of medicine at Harvard Medical School and a staff physician at Newton Wellesley Hospital in Newton, Massachusetts.

Other suggestions (that may have nothing to do with carbon dioxide) are to drink water very quickly or to swallow dry bread or crushed ice. For hiccups lasting longer than a day, see a physician.

Heartburn

This common problem, also known as indigestion, dyspepsia and gastroesophageal reflux, is a major source of usually minor discomfort for most of us. The symptoms, an uncomfortable burning in the chest or regurgitation, are caused when stomach acid washes upward into your esophagus. The lining of the esophagus has a low resistance to stomach acid, so you feel pain.

How that stomach acid gets into your esophagus is another story. Any one of several things can do it: a weak sphincter valve (the muscular door between stomach and esophagus that prevents digestive juices from backwashing), overeating, eating the wrong foods, stress, overweight and even pregnancy.

Under normal circumstances, the valve works fine.

But sometimes the valve is weak or pressure on the abdomen is too great, and those juices can get past the valve. The excess pressure can happen because your belly is larger than it should be or because you're pregnant. Overeating also puts more pressure on the valve.

Lying down also makes it easier for stomach acid to flow from stomach to esophagus. Nicotine, alcohol, chocolate and coffee (both decaf and regular) can cause that valve between your stomach and esophagus to relax. Some drugs, like tranquilizers and antispasmodics, may have the same effect. "So the worst thing is to have alcohol or coffee and a cigarette at bedtime," says Roger Gebhard, M.D., professor of medicine at the University of Minnesota and staff physician at the Minneapolis Veterans Administration Hospital.

The first and best defense, of course, is to prevent heartburn. "For many patients, losing some weight, loosening their belts or wearing suspenders may help," says Dr. Gebhard. "Stop or reduce smoking. Avoid alcohol, chocolate and coffee. It doesn't seem to matter whether the coffee has caffeine or not. Decaf produces the same symptoms. Try to avoid eating and lying down. Look at the drugs you're taking and talk them over with your physician. There may be less irritating substitutes."

Another approach to prevention is to raise the head of your bed. In this way, gravity can help hold the acid down in your stomach. But don't just use more pillows, says Dr. Gebhard—raise the whole headboard "so the head of the bed is raised six to eight inches. Many patients say that this technique was what stopped their symptoms over the long run."

And for those times when you aren't able to prevent heartburn, an over-the-counter antacid may extinguish the flames. Antacids do just what they say: They neutralize stomach acid. Most are effective for occasional heartburn, says Dr. Ginsburg, but you should know that there are different kinds. Some brands contain aluminum hydroxide, which may cause constipation. Others contain magnesium salts, which may cause diarrhea. The most popular, and most common, contain a combination of aluminum and magnesium, counteracting each ingredient's worst features. "Most people should look for a combination antacid," says Dr. Ginsburg. Some antacids contain calcium carbonate, and these may be the most effective.

Many antacids also contain sodium. If you have high blood pressure, Dr. Ginsburg says, your physician may steer you toward a low-sodium variety. Also consult your doctor if you're taking iron supplements or prescription medications like tetracycline or ciprofloxacin. Certain antacids may interfere with their absorption.

One old standby, sodium bicarbonate (baking soda), is generally not recommended. Says Dr. Gebhard, "Baking soda may relieve symptoms right away, but it raises the pH of the stomach so high that the stomach has a tendency to create more stomach acid. So in the long term, it is counterproductive, and it contains a lot of sodium."

If you take an antacid, Dr. Ginsburg suggests you follow these directions to maximize its effectiveness.

Liquid antacids generally work better than tablets, so take a liquid if it's convenient. Take the antacid an hour after eating, when the stomach is typically filled with acid, and then three hours later, since antacids usually aren't effective much longer than two hours. Take it again (assuming two or three hours have passed) at bedtime. For tablets, take two after eating and again at bedtime. Most important: A heart attack can sometimes be mistaken for heartburn and vice versa. So play it safe. If any of the following apply to you, call 911 (or the appropriate emergency number) right away, then call your doctor:

■ If the pressure, fullness, squeezing or pain in your chest persists despite taking antacids.

■ If the pressure is a new symptom.

■ If you have other symptoms along with the feeling of pressure in your chest, such as shortness of breath, sweating, nausea, dizziness, fainting, general weakness or pain radiating from your chest to your back, jaw or arms. When in doubt, make the call.

Nausea and Vomiting

When that old gastroenteritis has you in its spell, nausea and vomiting may make your life miserable. Unfortunately, these symptoms may be accompanied by diarrhea.

If a bug is the source of your queasiness, rest assured that the feeling will go away all by itself in a day or two. If it doesn't, advises Ralph Bernstein, M.D., chief of gastroenterology at Highland Hospital in Oakland, California, call your doctor.

The other causes of vomiting are legion: the morning sickness associated with pregnancy, motion sickness, a headache or migraine, food poisoning, some prescription medications and, of course, too much alcohol.

If you suspect that your queasiness is due to any of these, take heart. It will, in a word, pass. To ease your discomfort, Dr. Gebhard advises the following: Slowly replace lost fluids with water, weak tea or perhaps cola or ginger ale. (Some doctors advise that, if you use soda, you should let it go flat. All the carbonation is just another irritant. Avoid milk products.)

As the day progresses and your nausea eases, you can begin to put your system to the test. Try eating bland foods, such as dry toast and plain crackers. If they stay down, fine. If not, go back to liquids for a while.

Some OTC preparations may help, such as cola syrup. Bismuth-containing medications may also help.

Remember, if vomiting persists, or if it is accompanied by unexplained weight loss, abdominal pain or chest pain, by all means see your physician.

Lactose Intolerance

The bloating and diarrhea of lactose intolerance can be confused with the symptoms of other disorders, such as a sick stomach. But lactose intolerance is really quite different. People with a lactose intolerance are missing an enzyme called lactase that digests milk sugars (lactose) in the small intestine. "In everyday clinical practice, we see people who say that after they've had a glass of milk or a dish of ice cream, they've got to run for the bathroom," says Dr. Bernstein.

Lactose intolerance is particularly common in Asians, Jews, Native Americans and African-Americans. It affects an estimated 30 million Americans. If you suspect that your symptoms are linked to milk products in your diet, one way to check is through a lactose tolerance test. Ask your doctor about it.

If you are lactose intolerant, says Dr. Bernstein, "it's really more of a nuisance than anything else." Precisely how much milk is enough to set you off is very much an individual thing. One estimate is that about 30 percent of lactose-intolerant people start to feel symptoms after taking in about a quart of milk and dairy products. In an additional 30 to 40 percent, all it takes is a glassful. Generally, adds Dr. Bernstein, the small amount of milk found in a cookie isn't enough to provoke it.

So what to do if you are lactose intolerant? You can try taking one of the over-the-counter lactase supplements before consuming milk or other dairy products. Or try adding the supplements to the food or drinking one of the new milk products that already contain lactase. Some of Dr. Ginsburg's patients, although not all, have found that lactase helps.

Other tips:

Eat Yogurt ▶ Live cultures in yogurt are believed to produce lactase. These organisms may help your body digest the milk products in yogurt. Yogurt also contains a smaller amount of the offending lactose that causes your problems. And make it nonfat yogurt. Fat, true to its reputation, makes your digestive system sluggish and slows down emptying of stomach contents. There is also some evidence that eating yogurt before eating ice cream may help your body digest the lactose contained in that treat.

Say Cheese ▶ Try low-lactose cheeses. Most cheeses (except cottage cheese) have only a trace of lactose, especially hard cheeses like Parmesan and Romano.

Stick to Small Servings ▶ Begin with two to four ounces of dairy, to be on the safe side. Increase the serving size if you suffer no ill effects.

Drink Chocolate Milk ▶ Made with cocoa, that is. Pilot studies suggest that cocoa may ease symptoms of lactose intolerance.

Flatulence

Beans. Broccoli. Cabbage. All good foods, all essential elements of a balanced diet, all wonderful sources of fiber. And all, unfortunately, leading sources of intestinal gas. All three foods contain high quantities of nonabsorbable sugars. The bacteria in your intestines work to break the sugars down, creating large quantities of intestinal gas. Other foods, including brussels sprouts and cauliflower, may create a similar effect.

The best way to deal with gas is to not get it in the first place. But you don't want to steer clear of all high-fiber foods. You need them. Instead, try this strategy: Ease your system into high-fiber foods gradually, eating small amounts at first and increasing your intake as your body adjusts to them.

Another approach, useful for beans, is this: Rinse them until the water runs clear, then boil them for two minutes. Drain the water and replace it with fresh water. Let them stand overnight, or at least six hours. Drain them well. Add fresh water and cook according to your recipe.

The other option is to sprinkle your possibly gas-producing food with a substance called alpha-galactosidase (brand name Beano). Research suggests that this product may neutralize the effects of gas-producing foods.

Should you be burdened with gas in spite of all your precautions, some over-the-counter remedies might help you. Simethicone may give relief to some people. Other preparations containing activated charcoal may help absorb gas. But charcoal may interfere with the absorption of certain medications, so check with your physician first.

In addition to being caused by dietary factors, gas

may be the result of excessive air swallowing—the same kind that leads to belching. The air accumulates in the stomach, where some of it eventually makes its way to the colon. So any technique used to minimize too much air-swallowing (discussed above) may also help prevent gas.

Constipation

Perhaps 10 to 20 percent of all otherwise healthy people suffer from chronic constipation, says Dr. Gebhard.

Regularity, unfortunately, is often in the eye of the beholder. Some people believe they're constipated if they don't have a bowel movement every day. But, says Dr. Gebhard, that's not necessarily true. Some people normally have three movements a day, while others may have three a week. Nevertheless, some people go to a lot of trouble, to the point of becoming dependent on laxatives, in the mistaken belief that they absolutely must have a bowel movement daily. Generally, you're considered constipated if more than three days go by without a bowel movement, according to the National Digestive Diseases Information Clearinghouse.

The causes are numerous, including, but not limited to, inadequate fiber in the diet, poor intake of fluids, insufficient exercise and the use of certain OTC and prescription medications containing aluminum (such as antacids), antidepressants, antispasmodics, tranquilizers, iron pills and anticonvulsants.

Among older adults in particular, inactivity and poor diet are the most likely causes. Stress and changing dietary habits because of travel can also contribute to that stopped-up feeling.

For prevention of constipation, an adequate daily intake of fiber is essential—about 20 to 35 grams a day for most people. Unprocessed bran, whole-wheat bread and that old standby, prune juice, are highly recommended. Drinking six to eight glasses of water a day should also help, as should moderate amounts of daily exercise.

But if you become constipated in spite of all your best efforts, here's what to do. If you feel you need a laxative, start with one of the mildest ones first—that is, a bulk-forming fiber supplement for three to five days. If that doesn't work, you might try a liquid laxative. If you still get no relief after a day or two, check with your doctor.

There are several types of laxatives that may do the trick, but they all do different things. Some are stimulants that trigger contractions in the intestines. Others are known as osmotic laxatives, and these bring more water into the colon. Stool softeners do just what they say, and you can guess what lubricants do. Your doctor will recommend the one that should work best for you.

It's important not to use stimulant laxatives longer than one to two weeks without a doctor's supervision, says Dr. Gebhard. "The colon may lose its ability to function normally without that crutch," he says. Then you have a whole new set of problems to deal with, including establishing regularity again.

At the onset of a bout with constipation, if you experience other symptoms, such as abdominal pain or fever, consult your physician.

Diarrhea

There are between 50 and 100 known causes of diarrhea, from serious illnesses like cancer to stage fright. The three most common are viral infections, bacterial infections and parasites, such as the turista variety encountered in overseas travels.

For most of us, an occasional bout of diarrhea may bring discomfort and watery stools for a day or two and then come to an end. Should diarrhea come your way, your most immediate concern is to replace the fluid that you're losing. A second concern is not to aggravate your already irritated colon with foods it can't handle.

"Stay away from heavy foods," says Dr. Bernstein. "Avoid milk products. Consume only clear soups and other liquids. Cola drinks are okay and may actually decrease the amount of diarrhea you have." Try the BRAT diet: bananas, rice, applesauce and dry toast in small quantities. If they stay with you, fine. If they don't, go back to just liquids for a while.

Diarrhea is your body's way of ridding itself of infection or parasites. So the best bet is to wait it out before trying medication. If, however, you need relief so you can go about your daily routine, you can try over-the-counter remedies. Among the most common treatments are the so-called adsorbent diarrhea remedies containing attapulgite, methylcellulose or psyllium. These absorb water and irritants in the bowel, producing more formed bowel movements.

More recently, the Food and Drug Administration has permitted the over-the-counter sale of certain medications that contain small amounts of a narcotic that slows down the muscles in the bowel, so movements pass more slowly. These are considered most effective, though adsorbents are milder. Don't take adsorbents along with the narcotics. They could work too well, obstructing the bowel. And don't take the narcotic medications for more than two days. Antidiarrheals containing bismuth salicylate may be helpful for traveler's diarrhea.

If your diarrhea continues longer than two days, consult your doctor. Also call your physician, advises Dr. Bernstein, if you have any of the following symptoms: fever, nausea or vomiting, or blood in the stools.

Put Your Back Pain Behind You 10

Using yoga to control sacroiliac pain and sciatica.

By Mary Pullig Schatz, M.D.

75

Many people confuse sacroiliac pain with sciatica because the two conditions share a similar symptom—a dull ache or stabbing pain between the lower back and the hip on one side. However, the causes of the pain are quite different.

With sacroiliac problems, the pain is felt on either side of the base of the spine, in the sacroiliac joints. With sciatica, the pain is felt deep in the buttock in the soft tissues near the sacroiliac (SI) joint and extends down the leg along the course of the sciatic nerve.

The key to finding relief is first to identify which pain has you in its grip and second to understand its causes. Only then can you take action to correct the underlying problem through a carefully designed program of gentle yoga exercises.

Sacroiliac Pain

Sacroiliac pain is usually experienced as a dull ache in the bones above the buttock on one side. But because the nerves in that region are not very specific, pain caused by the SI joint can also be experienced in the groin, back thigh and lower abdomen. Usually there is no numbness or tingling when someone has this problem, but there may be a dull, heavy feeling in the leg.

The joints of the bones that form the pelvis, unlike those of the arms, legs and spine, are held firmly together by ligaments to give great stability and to allow little movement. The SI joints are on either side of the base of the spine.

Sacroiliac pain results when slight pelvic rotation, or torsion, creates abnormal stresses on the ligaments that join the two bones together. Golf, racket sports and ballet dancing can cause pelvic torsion, placing rotational stress on the sacroiliac joint. Asymmetry of the pelvic bones or unequal leg or hamstring length can also cause SI pain. For instance, if the pelvis is tilted to one side, the forces on the two SI joints will be different. Hypermobile sacroiliac joints often lead to SI pain in pregnant women due to the hormone relaxin, which relaxes a woman's ligaments in preparation for childbirth.

76

The source of sacroiliac pain is usually a misalignment of the pelvis. To begin to correct SI pain, you must first be aware that asymmetry exists and that any asymmetrical posture (like sitting with your legs crossed or standing with your weight on one foot) will make the problem worse.

Therapeutic exercise for pain in the sacroiliac area is directed at stretching the hamstrings, buttocks and lower back muscles (which frequently go into spasm when there are SI problems), strengthening all the muscles of the hip girdle to provide support for the pelvis and strengthening the abdominal muscles to support the front of the spine.

In order to perform therapeutic exercises for SI pain, however, you must first know which way the pelvis is rotated. If the pelvis is rotated to the right, the right SI joint will protrude more prominently than the left. Similarly, when the pelvis is rotated to the left, the left SI joint will be more prominent.

Sacral Rock ▶ Lie on your back on a bare or thinly carpeted floor, with your knees bent and your feet parallel on the floor a few inches away from your buttocks. If you do not have an uncarpeted floor, place a hardcover book or thin board (less than ½ inch thick) under your sacrum. Place a rolled towel for neck support behind your neck and a head pad (folded towel) under your head. Keep these props handy, as you will need them again.

Keeping your knees together and your feet on the floor, move your knees slowly to the right six to eight inches, and then back to the starting position. Then move your knees slowly to the left and then back. Repeat this at least ten times. Notice any asymmetry in the right and left sides of the sacrum during the rocking action. If one SI joint seems to push into the floor more prominently than the other, the pelvis is rotated to that side.

Note: Do not practice this pose during the second half of pregnancy.

Supine Cobbler's Pose ▶ Lie on your back, with appropriate head and neck padding. Place the soles of your feet together, with your knees bent. Have your heels as close to your sitting bones as comfortably possible.

While breathing quietly, rock your pelvis slowly in a circle over the sacrum, pressing along its outer edges.

Breathe softly and quietly. Imagine a circle around your sacrum and move the weight of your pelvis smoothly around the periphery of that circle. Go around the circle clockwise twice and then counterclockwise twice. Repeat for a total of two to four sets.

By moving your pelvis in a circle, you can massage the sacrum and determine additional information about the symmetry of the SI joints. With persistence, over many months you can also help the protruding SI joint gradually slip back into alignment. This is also an abdominal-muscle strengthener.

Note: Do not practice this pose during the second half of pregnancy.

Knee to Chest, Extend Other Leg ▶ This pose will help you correct pelvic torsion. Lie on your back with both knees bent and your feet on the floor. Use appropriate head and neck padding. Repeat the Sacral Rock and once again note which SI joint is more prominent. If your pelvis is rotated, one SI joint will feel as though it is protruding more into the floor; the other will feel more concave or hollow.

Bend the knee on the side of the more protuberant SI joint toward your chest and hold it there, with your hands holding the back of your thigh (not your knee). Straighten the other leg and lift it three inches from the floor. Stretch out through the heel and then slowly place the leg back on the floor.

Draw the bent leg closer to your chest. Lift the straight leg three inches from the floor, extend it out to the side as far as it will go—for most people, one to two feet—and slowly lower it to the floor. Allow your pelvis to rock to that side as you lower your leg. (The weight of the leg helps to derotate the pelvis.) Then return the leg to the starting position. Once again, draw the bent leg closer to the chest, raise the straight leg three inches from the floor, extend it out to the side and then set it down.

Then place both feet on the floor with your knees bent and repeat the Sacral Rock to see if the position of the SI joints has changed. If there is a decrease in prominence or tenderness of the protuberant side and a more normal (less caved-in) feeling on the other side, repeat the exercise, again drawing the knee on the side of the more protuberant SI joint toward your chest.

If this adjustment does not make a correction, then try it with a small weight (such as a two-pound bag of beans) held on your outstretched thigh by an elastic bandage. This will provide more leverage.

If this exercise exaggerates the SI protuberance, try reversing legs and see if that helps. If you can't correct the pelvic torsion, practice the Sacral Rock and the Supine Cobbler's Pose for a few months, then try this exercise again.

Note: This is an unusual exercise in that it is not repeated on both sides; only the side that gives correction is practiced. Do not practice this pose during the second half of pregnancy.

Sciatica

Characteristically, this pain starts in the buttock and extends down the rear of the thigh and lower leg to the sole of the foot and along the outer side of the lower leg to the top of the foot. Pain may also be felt in the lower back.

Several nerve roots leave the spinal cord, exit through holes in the sacrum and combine to form the sciatic nerve, which passes between layers of the deep buttock muscles and then into the deep muscles of the back of the thigh.

A primary cause of sciatica is a herniated or bulging lower lumbar intervertebral disk that compresses one of the nerve roots before it joins the sciatic nerve. Sometimes irritation of a branch of the sciatic nerve in the leg can be so severe as to set up a reflex pain reaction involving the entire length of the nerve. For example, if the nerve is pinched or irritated near the knee, you may feel the pain in the hip and buttock.

Another cause of sciatica is the piriformis syndrome. The piriformis muscle extends from the side of the sacrum to the top of the thighbone at the hip joint, passing over the sciatic nerve en route. When a short or tight piriformis is stretched, it can compress and irritate the sciatic nerve.

Because the piriformis muscle acts to rotate the leg outward, people who habitually stand with their toes turned out often develop piriformis syndrome, as do runners and cyclists, who overuse and understretch the piriformis muscle.

To alleviate sciatica, you must deal with its basic cause. If you have a herniated disk or the bulging disk condition is severe, disk surgery might be required. If, however, the source of your sciatica is a slightly bulging disk or pressure from a short, tight piriformis muscle, the most effective course of treatment is simply to do some carefully designed yoga stretches.

Piriformis Stretch ▶ This is designed to place the piriformis in a stretched position in order to cause it to lengthen over time. Therefore, in someone with sciatic pain due to a short piriformis, this pose will re-create that pain. It is of utmost importance that the pose be adjusted so that you feel a minimum amount of discomfort; the muscle should be encouraged to lengthen by gentle stretching. If it is stretched too vigorously, the pain will be unbearable and the muscle will go into spasm, further worsening the condition.

Sit on the corner of a neatly folded blanket four to six inches high, with your knees bent and your feet flat on the floor in front of you. Take your right foot under your left knee and place it on its side on the floor next to your left buttock. The outside of your right leg should then be resting on the floor with the knee centered in front of your body. Then place the sole of your left foot on the floor next to the outside of your right thigh. Feel your weight resting equally on both sitting bones. From this base, allow your spine to lengthen upward as you gently lift your breastbone.

Stabilize your trunk by holding your left knee with both hands. If your left foot won't reach the floor by your right thigh or if the stretch in your left buttock is too intense, place your left foot next to or in front of your right knee instead.

If the stretch is still too intense or you feel radiating pain down your leg (indicating sciatic nerve irritation), raise the height of the padding beneath your buttocks to decrease the intensity of the stretch to a tolerable level. If you don't feel any stretch in your left buttock, gently pull your left knee across your body toward the right side of your chest.

Stay in the pose for 20 seconds to several minutes. Then repeat on the other side. Do two to four sets. As your piriformis muscles stretch out over a period of months, gradually decrease the height of your blankets until you can sit on the floor.

Double-Duty Relief

Whether your pain is caused by sacroiliac problems or an irritated sciatic nerve, any of the following yoga exercises will be therapeutic for you.

If you have sciatica due to a tight piriformis or buttock pain due to piriformis spasm, practice the Piriformis Stretch at least once a day along with any or all of these basic exercises. If you have pelvic torsion, first do the preceding corrective exercises so that you start the following exercises in good alignment.

Supine Pelvic Tilt ▶ Lie on your back with your knees bent and your feet parallel on the floor. Place your arms comfortably at your sides, palms up. Then place your head pad under your head and your neck-support roll under your neck.

Inhale into your chest and abdomen. Let your chest and belly expand. As you exhale, move your navel toward the floor. This action will take your lower back toward the floor as well. Inhale again into your abdomen; on an exhalation, again press your navel and lower back toward the floor. At the same time, press your shoulders, elbows and the back of your head into the floor. Keep your legs entirely passive. Repeat slowly at least ten times. Work toward being able to hold the position for 10 to 20 seconds.

Roll to your side and then sit up.

Imagine your spine assuming a more normal configuration. Explore the feelings in the muscles called on to produce this action. Realize that by pressing down with the shoulders and elbows, you are keeping your shoulders from rounding and your chest from collapsing as you move your navel toward the floor.

An important first step in reeducating your posture, this exercise teaches awareness of chest alignment and its relationship to the position of the pelvis and the lumbar spine. It also begins to strengthen the abdominal muscles, an important step in creating a healthy back.

Note: If you have a flat lumbar curve, do this pose with a folded towel (one inch thick by four inches wide) behind your waist to support your lumbar curve. If you have spondylolysis or spondylolisthesis, this is an important pose for you. Do not practice this pose during the second half of pregnancy.

Yoga Sit-Ups ▶ Lie on your back with your calves resting on a chair seat. Your hips as well as your knees should be bent at about a 90-degree angle. Cross your arms in front of your chest and place your hands on your shoulders. To avoid neck strain, do not place your hands on your neck!

If you want more challenge, lightly hold each earlobe or cross your arms behind your head and touch each shoulder blade with the opposite hand. Do not place your hands on your neck. Inhale. Begin a long, slow exhalation, during which you:

■ Tilt the pelvis as described in the preceding pose, so your lower back moves to the floor as you flatten your abdomen.

■ Raise your shoulders six to ten inches off the floor, no higher.

■ Lower your right shoulder to touch the floor and raise it back up.

■ Continue exhaling as you lower your trunk to the floor.

■ Inhale. Then, on a long, slow exhalation, repeat the preceding sequence, this time lowering and raising your left shoulder. Visualize your abdominal muscles getting stronger as you use them to lift your trunk. Repeat the sequence with proper breathing until your abdominal muscles feel warm. Then do one or two more and stop. Roll to the side and use the strength of your arms to push yourself into a seated position.

Having the hips flexed at about 90 degrees prevents injury to the lumbar spine. Lifting the trunk while exhaling places the abdominals in a shortened position for strengthening, preventing you from ending up with strong but "puffed out" (protruding) abdominal muscles less capable of lumbar support. Lifting straight up strengthens the midline abdominal muscles. Lowering and lifting each shoulder strengthens the other abdominal muscles. The abdomen should not bulge out but should feel flatter and wider during this exercise.

Safe strengthening of the abdominal muscles is crucial to proper positioning of the pelvis and maintenance of a healthy lumbar curve.

Note: Do not hold your breath during any part of these exercises. If you have a flat lumbar curve, use your lumbar pad to create and support a more natural curve during these exercises. If you have spondylolysis or spondylolisthesis, these are important poses for you. Do not practice this pose during the second half of pregnancy.

Supine Knee-Chest Twist ▶ Lie on your back with your neck-support roll and head pad in place. Place your arms out to each side, palms up. Bend both knees and draw them together toward your chest. Inhale, and on the exhalation, let both knees slowly and gently down to the floor on one side of your body. Rest them there for 30 to 60 seconds. Inhale, and on the exhalation, slowly lift your knees back to the starting position. Repeat on the other side. Do three to five sets.

Note: If you have spondylolysis or spondylolisthesis, this is an important pose for you. Do not practice this pose during the second half of pregnancy.

Easy Bridge Pose ▶ Lie on your back with a neatly folded blanket, two inches thick, under your shoulders and your knees bent. Place your feet parallel, flat on the floor, with your heels close to your buttocks and hip-width apart. Have your thighs parallel and your arms at your sides, palms up.

On an exhalation, press your lower back into the floor by using the abdominal muscles to draw the pubic bone toward the breastbone, tilting the pelvis. Hold this position during the next inhalation.

On the next exhalation, begin to lift your buttocks by pressing your feet firmly into the floor while maintaining a strong pelvic tilt. Lift your buttocks six to eight inches off the floor, keeping your breathing relaxed and your eyes looking down. Maintain a firm pressure of your shoulders and elbows against the floor.

To keep your thighs from separating, press evenly into the bottoms of your feet. Resist the tendency for the weight to shift to the outer edges of the feet by pressing down with the inner heels. Keep your chest from going down by moving your breastbone toward your head as much as you can. Your knees should stay hip-width apart. Keep your shoulders, jaw and face relaxed.

Return to the starting position on an exhalation. As you lower your hips, keep your pubic bone moving toward the breastbone and your buttocks sweeping toward the backs of your knees. Repeat three to six times.

Breathe smoothly, quietly and gently, coordinating the breath with the pose. Move only on an exhalation. Do not hold your breath.

If you can't raise your buttocks six to eight inches, don't despair. Concentrate on drawing your pubic bone toward your breastbone and on pressing your feet firmly into the floor. From there, lift your buttocks any amount; even ½ inch allows you to benefit from the pose.

This pose strengthens the buttock muscles, the hamstrings and the abdominals. It stretches the hip flexors, corrects both flat and increased lumbar curves and improves rounded shoulders.

Note: Do not practice these poses during the second half of pregnancy.

One Leg Up, One Leg Out ▶ Find a place, such as a doorway, where you can stretch one leg up the wall and stretch the other straight on the floor.

Sit with your right side close to the wall. Then, supporting your trunk with your arms, lie down and extend your right leg up the wall. Support your neck and head with your neck-support roll and head pad. Keep your left leg bent, with the foot on the floor. Let your arms rest easily at your sides. Adjust the position of your buttocks so that your right leg can be fully straightened and your sacrum can rest solidly on the floor. If you can't completely straighten your right leg, move your buttocks away from the wall until you can straighten your leg while maintaining a comfortable hamstring stretch. The feeling in the hamstrings should be a gentle muscle stretch, not overstretch pain.

Once the buttocks are positioned, slowly stretch out your left leg. If your lower back hurts when your left leg is outstretched on the floor, place a rolled blanket behind your knee so your lower back is comfortable.

Repeat on the other side. Hold each side for two to five minutes.

For a greater challenge, bend the knee of the raised leg and then actively straighten the leg as you pull back on the toes and stretch up through the heel. This will intensify the stretch, so go easy!

This position allows you to stretch the hamstrings of one leg and the hip flexors of the other leg.

Note: If you have a flat lumbar curve, use your lumbar pad. If these poses aggravate your sciatica, try moving your buttocks farther from the wall. If that does not eliminate the pain, skip them for now and work on other poses for a month before trying it again. If you have scoliosis, spondylolysis or spondylolisthesis, these are important poses for you. Do not practice these poses during the second half of pregnancy. If you notice an asymmetry in hamstring flexibility, you may also have pelvic torsion, caused by uneven pulling of the hamstrings on the pelvis.

85

11

Say "Adios" to Allergies

Don't be a slave to these seasonal miseries.

When warm weather comes, it's the survival of the fittest. Who's going to win—you or your hay fever? Well, no matter how much sneezing and dripping and blowing and suffering you did last year, this year will be different. That's because the American College of Allergy and Immunology has devised this survival guide for the upcoming allergy season.

When it comes to hay fever—a problem known to doctors as allergic rhinitis—you need all the help you can get. So here's some intelligence information on the enemy (pollen, especially ragweed) and a battle plan that can put you on the offensive.

What You're Up Against

That little 40-micron-diameter ragweed pollen—the smaller the pollen, the more potent it is—is only looking for a friend, but too often it finds your nose. And there it sets off a remarkable chain of immune-system chemical events that can best be described as a cascade—one thing leads to another, tumbling along, gaining in speed and force, until your nose, eyes and throat are the body's version of Niagara Falls.

"When we breathe in an allergen, the first reaction is from the mast cells," says allergist Charles Banov, M.D., clinical professor of internal medicine at the Medical University of South Carolina in Charleston. These large immune-system cells contain histamine, a chemical that causes immediate swelling and production of mucus in the nose, sinuses and eyes. "The allergen that has attached itself to the mast cell's membrane also disrupts the membrane, starting a process that leads to the production of some very strong substances that cause allergy symptoms," Dr. Banov says.

One of these chemicals attracts a type of white blood cell that sticks to the cells in the lining of the nose and releases a protein that's toxic to them. "The protein literally shreds the lining cells, and when the cells peel off into the airway, it's like taking bricks out of a brick wall," Dr. Banov says. The hole exposes nerve endings that give off a whole slew of other inflammatory chemicals, which in turn attract still more immune-system cells, which themselves churn out even more inflammatory substances, such as interferons and interleukins. These chemicals go to work on the poor mast cells, and 5 to 12 hours later—after your first bout of sneezing and sniffling—a second wave of symptoms strikes.

All it took was a good hit of tiny ragweed pollen, and now you've got a phenomenally complex stew of immune-system chemicals and a smorgasbord of symptoms. And it doesn't stop at your nose. It can make your eyes itch, plug up your eustachian tubes, send mucus dripping down your throat and fill your sinuses to the point that they are set up for infection. And, if you have asthma, it can trigger an attack.

Why you? Why not the guy down the street with the ragweed lawn? Because he doesn't have your genes and your sensitivity threshold. Oxford University scientists have narrowed the search to one of three or four genes on the eleventh chromosome, says Sandra Gawchik, D.O., co-director of the Division of Allergy at Crozer-Chester Medical Center in Chester, Pennsylvania.

You inherited the ability to produce an antibody called immunoglobulin E, or IgE, which reacts to allergens and starts the chemical cascade, says allergist David Tinkelman, M.D., clinical professor of pediatrics in the Department of Allergy and Immunology at the Medical College of Georgia in Augusta. "People who don't have the IgE antibody don't have the ability to respond to the allergens in pollen and mold," he says.

Yet even with IgE, allergies are not inevitable. Some people with IgE never develop allergies. It all depends on your own allergy threshold. Some children start out with allergy symptoms, lose them as they go through the hormonal changes of puberty and get them

87

back in adulthood, "sometimes following a hormonal change as in pregnancy, or maybe after a significant viral illness that changes the body's immune system," Dr. Tinkelman says.

Other IgE people don't show allergies until a period of emotional stress descends, says allergist Gilbert Barkin, M.D., past president of the American College of Allergy and Immunology. "Although I tested positive for allergies, I never actually had allergies until my threshold was lowered by the stress of my mother's major illness," Dr. Barkin says.

Over the years, allergies tend to follow a script, says Edward O'Connell, M.D., professor of pediatrics, allergy and immunology at Mayo Medical School in Rochester, Minnesota. "If you wrote a play about someone with an allergy, in act one there is no problem, in act two it looks like there is a problem, in act three the problem is worsening, in act four it plateaus, and in act five it declines." Once you reach age 55 or so, allergies usually subside as your immune system's efficiency begins to decline.

Hay fever is not an abnormality, Dr. O'Connell says. It hits up to 22 percent of the population, making it the sixth most prevalent chronic condition in the country, outranking even heart disease. It's no wonder that science has devised many ways to handle it.

First-Line Defense and Offense

The overall strategy in fighting allergic rhinitis is not to do more than you have to. That means you have to decide how bad your hay fever is. If you think it's tolerable, you can treat yourself (with your family physician's help, if need be). If it's ruining your life, you need to see an allergist. Here's what you can do if your condition isn't serious yet (although some of the following is definitely a part of any serious anti-hay-fever approach).

88

Be Prepared ▶ The main weapon of self-treatment is an over-the-counter antihistamine. All antihistamines work the same way: They block the effects of histamine.

No histamine, no runny nose or itchy eyes. But you have to be a good tactician to get the most out of them, says Fort Worth allergist/immunologist Susan Rudd Wynn, M.D. "You have to take them before your exposure to allergens," she says. "Don't wait until you're miserable or losing sleep. During your allergy season, have antihistamines in your system 24 hours a day. Many people don't want to take medication unless they absolutely have to, but sleep deprivation is one of the worst aspects of hay fever."

Experiment ▶ An antihistamine that works for your friend may not work for you, Dr. Wynn says. One person's perfect pill may be your dud. If it doesn't work, try another.

Switch ▶ After taking an antihistamine for a while, you may find it doesn't work as well as it used to. That's because people often build up tolerance to OTC antihistamines, Dr. O'Connell says. "Until the new prescription drugs came along, we used to be changing people over to different medications every couple of weeks because the OTCs wouldn't be effective any longer." So be prepared to find a new drug.

Use Decongestants ▶ Main side effect of antihistamines is drowsiness, which is the main reason people don't like to take them, Dr. Wynn says. And though they dry you up, antihistamines don't unplug you. That's where the combination drugs come in handy—they contain drying, nap-inducing antihistamines and unplugging, stimulating decongestants. Coffee might seem like a good antidrowsy drug, "but antihistamines and caffeine work at different places in the brain," Dr. Wynn says, "so you could end up drowsy and crabby."

But use decongestants wisely. While they're generally safe, decongestants can be tricky. Their stimulant effect can keep you up at night, make you jittery and irritable during the day and suppress your appetite, Dr. Wynn says. To get through the day fully awake, you may want to take a combination drug and at night switch to an antihistamine-only drug, she says. Although decongestants are safe enough to be sold without a prescription, if you have heart problems or high blood pressure, you probably shouldn't take them, Dr. Wynn says. Check with your doctor first.

Get a Prescription ▶ If your hay fever is regular and short-lived—September is Sneeze Month, for example—and you don't like OTC medications, ask your family doctor for a nonsedating antihistamine available only by prescription. "They're far better tolerated than the traditional antihistamines because far less of them reaches the brain," Dr. O'Connell says. They act just as quickly and work just as well as the OTC preparations, he says, and are also available as combination antihistamine/decongestants.

Snort a Snootful ▶ Nasal sprays can work wonders, but stick with the prescription-only cortisone-steroid nasal sprays, Dr. O'Connell advises. The cortisone sprays are vast improvements over the OTC sprays and well worth the visit to your doctor. "They've been a boon," Dr. O'Connell says. "Habituation to the OTC sprays is common, and there's a vicious rebound effect, so your nose gets worse than ever. With a cortisone spray, you don't develop tolerance, you don't get the rebound phenomenon, and the side effects are close to zero even after years of use."

Although these sprays take four to five days to start working, they're something you can use preventively, they work very well together with antihistamines, and they don't have the side effects of oral decongestants. The only time you should use the OTC sprays is when you are so stuffed up you can't sleep or to open your nose enough so the cortisone spray can get in, Dr. Wynn says.

Cromolyn nasal sprays are not steroids, and they're not as effective, Dr. O'Connell says, but if you want to avoid the steroids, cromolyn can be helpful. "The drawback is that cromolyn takes two to three weeks to kick in. During that time you're miserable, and pretty soon your allergy season is over anyway," he says. So cromolyn is a medication you want to start taking a few weeks before your allergy season hits.

Avoid Alcohol ▶ "Alcohol is a vasodilator, so if you're already a little stopped up, even if it's not noticeable, alcohol can cause you to become noticeably congested," Dr. Wynn says. "And you get a dangerous sedative effect if you mix antihistamines with alcohol," which is why every antihistamine package label warns against it.

Avoid Smoke ▶ "Smoking can trigger hay fever, and many people, when they stop smoking, begin to realize how many, or how few, nasal problems they have," Dr. O'Connell says.

Watch the Pollen Counts ▶ Use the pollen counts issued by the media to keep track of when your pollen season starts so you know when to start your avoidance tactics (or to start taking your medication), Dr. Wynn advises. Generally, the counts aren't too good for planning day-to-day activities, however, because by the time you see them, they're a couple of days old, she says. And by the end of the season they're not much good at all because of what's called the priming effect: "Your nose has been bombarded all season, it's inflamed and primed for firing, so it may take only 1 to 10 percent of the pollen dose it took earlier to make your nose go off," she says.

Air Condition Your Bedroom ▶ And switch on the air conditioner at night. Keep the windows closed. "Some of my patients would turn on the air conditioning, but on mild days they would also keep the windows open, totally defeating the purpose of filtering the air," Dr. O'Connell says.

Air Condition Your Car ▶ And keep the windows closed at all times.

Keep Your Air Conditioners Clean ▶ "Molds can grow in an air conditioner, so you have to clean the filter and water pan periodically," says St. Louis allergist

Raymond Slavin, M.D., director of the Division of Allergy and Immunology at St. Louis University School of Medicine.

Keep Your Lawn Mowed Short ▶ This ensures that it doesn't have a chance to pollinate. Don't mow the lawn yourself, and stay inside during neighborhood lawn-mowing day. If you do have to mow the lawn or rake the leaves, wear a pollen mask or scarf over your nose and mouth. And don't lie on the grass or take a stroll through fields of weeds.

Give Up Sun-Drying Your Clothes ▶ "They pick up pollen out of the air," Dr. Gawchik says, and when you bury your face in that shirt you get a snootful of pollen.

Reconsider Moving ▶ Moving isn't worth it. "There's no place that is the worst for pollen allergy, and there's no place that's totally free of pollen," says allergist William Storms, M.D., associate professor of medicine at the University of Colorado School of Medicine in Denver. "Thirty or 40 years ago, Phoenix and Tucson had very low pollen counts, so people moved there for their allergies. But they decided they wanted grass lawns and sprinkler systems and trees, so now pollen and mold counts are higher than they've ever been."

The other problem with moving is that if you're allergic one place, you'll probably become allergic anyplace. "If you're living in Colorado and you're allergic to tumbleweed, you could move to the East Coast to get away from it," Dr. Storms says. "So you get better, but probably not for long, because you can develop allergies to new things—but you won't know that for two or three years."

Stay Inside between 5 and 10 A.M. ▶ That's when pollinating plants are at their most active.

Avoid Pollution ▶ "Pollutants definitely aggravate allergies," Dr. Storms says. "Your nose and eyes and sinuses are more sensitive to everything because of your hay fever. 'Everything' includes air pollution, cigarette smoke, certain perfumes and hair sprays, bug sprays, oven cleaners and, interestingly enough, the fragrance of laundry detergent. You can walk down the laundry detergent aisle in the supermarket and sneeze like crazy."

Seeing an Allergist

"One of the biggest complications of hay fever is the miseries one feels," Dr. O'Connell says. "Food doesn't taste right, you can't sleep well, you feel lousy." If you're at that stage and your doctor is telling you there's nothing more to be done, you should see a board-certified allergist. And there are ways to get the most out of your allergist.

Go Prepared ▶ "If you write down your symptoms at home before you visit the allergist, you're prepared and not as intimidated as you might be otherwise," Dr. Gawchik says.

Take Your Spouse ▶ "He or she may have an insight you don't have, know symptoms you're not aware of," she says. "And a lot of people are embarrassed that they might have too many complaints, so they don't tell the doctor everything. The more you tell, the more likely it is that the allergist can solve the problem."

Expect the Visit to Take a While ▶ The doctor should give you time and ask you a lot of questions. Your first visit could take 45 minutes to an hour, and that's not in the reception room. If you don't get plenty of the doctor's time, find another doctor, Dr. Gawchik advises. "I want to figure out what your problem is, what we need to do so that you can have a normal lifestyle and what medicines are suited to you. I want to know when your symptoms first developed, how long you've had them, how they affect you, what things seem to trigger your problems, whether you see a specific pattern and what you want from the doctor," she says.

The doctor should also ask what other medications you're taking, since beta-agonists, oral contraceptives and thyroid hormones can exacerbate or imitate allergy symptoms. "I want to sort of tune you up like a piano, until you can be as symptom free as possible," Dr. Gawchik says.

Ask Questions ▶ "It's important that you ask questions, too," she says. "And if you don't understand an answer, ask again, or ask the doctor to write it down for you, to recommend a book to read, to tell you what the medication is, how it works, what the side effects are, how it interacts with other medications you might be on."

After taking your personal history, the doctor should examine your nose and sinuses, looking for conditions that can cause symptoms similar to hay fever—a deviated septum, nasal polyps, adenoid hypertrophy or, rarely, cancer.

The allergist's war chest is deep, and your allergy armor can be custom-tailored to fit. The weapons range from avoidance to prescription medications to allergy testing to immunotherapy. But before your antiallergy program can be customized, you usually have to be tested. Skin or blood tests can tell you what you're allergic to, and then you and your doctor can decide whether the avoidance strategy is enough for you or if you need immunotherapy.

"The skin test measures the IgE antibody response to an allergen placed on your arm or back and then pricked through the skin," Dr. Tinkelman says. "If you have the IgE antibody to that particular allergen, you react with a release of histamine, which causes a red dot in about 20 minutes. It's the most accurate way to determine what you're allergic to."

"The new techniques are not at all painful," Dr. Slavin says. "It's not like getting an injection. Now there's a multitest device, a board with eight skin-test sites on it. You just load up the board with allergens, turn it over and press it on the arm and you have eight skin tests at once." One problem with skin testing is that it's so sensitive that it can produce false-positive readings, Dr. Barkin says.

94

A less sensitive test is the RAST, a blood test for your IgE's reaction to allergens. If the thought of several needle pricks is just too much—as it is for many people—or if you have skin problems or a rash, you can get your blood drawn once, and that's it. A RAST can give false-negative results, Dr. Barkin says, and there are fewer allergen tests that can be used with it.

Immunotherapy: The Last Resort

"Some people with allergies often don't realize that they have as much of a problem as they actually have," Dr. Storms says. "One lady I was treating told me, 'I'm doing so much better, these medicines are just remarkable and my allergies are gone.' Then she sneezed and blew her nose.

"I said, 'That may be true, but today you must be having some problems.' She said, 'Oh, no, this is normal. Before I came to see you, I had to have a box of tissues in every room in my house, and I used four boxes a week. Now one box lasts me two weeks.' So I asked her, 'How many boxes do you think a normal person would use?' She said, 'Well, about half a box a week is normal.' And I said, 'No, zero is normal.' A person with allergies gets used to having those symptoms and thinks they're just part of being human. Instead, you should see it as a problem that can be solved."

That woman probably is a good candidate for immunotherapy. And so are you, if you're having hay fever for several months a year, if OTC drugs, avoidance and prescription medications don't seem to work, even though you're taking them all the time, and if you're getting secondary problems, such as sinus infections or asthma attacks.

Formerly called desensitization, immunotherapy is a series of injections of the allergens that affect you, "in very minute quantities," Dr. Tinkelman says. "You're actually changing the immune system to keep it from releasing histamine. It's not exactly known how this works, but we think it's building up a different kind of antibody called a blocking antibody—immunoglobulin G, or IgG—that prevents the IgE from releasing the histamine." (IgG is the immune system's first-line antibody, sent to fight infection until the immune system learns what the invader is and releases a more specific antibody.)

Immunotherapy has repeatedly been shown to work, Dr. O'Connell says. You begin with low doses so as not to overload your system and gradually work up to high doses, he says. "Immunotherapy at present works only in high doses," he says. "Low and moderate doses have been shown not to work."

New research is finding that oral immunotherapy may also help, Dr. O'Connell says. "The latest concept is that oral is not as good as injections but is better than a placebo," he says.

Immunotherapy does have a few drawbacks: It's slow, it's not cheap and, rarely, it can cause anaphylactic shock in people who have asthma. The reaction risk is one reason that you should get immunotherapy only from a board-certified allergist.

"Once you're in the middle of the season and you're having lots of problems, it's too late for immunotherapy to do anything," Dr. Tinkelman says. "It takes too long to build up your blocking antibodies"—the minimum is three months—"so your doctor may say, 'Once allergy season is over, let's start with immunotherapy to prevent this happening again next year.'"

Once you've started the therapy, your immunity to the allergens should build up over the next year or two. "You probably can mount the protection you need over three to five years, starting out with one shot a week and then decreasing to one a month or one every six weeks," Dr. Wynn says. "And even if your allergy is only seasonal, you need to continue the shots all year."

How long does immunotherapy last? "You probably don't have to get the shots for the rest of your life," Dr. Wynn says. But there have been no good studies of what happens when people stop immunotherapy. Some studies have shown that some people continue their immunity, others have mild allergic symptoms, and still others have complete relapses. But a controlled study reported in 1988 found that people continued their resistance to allergens after immunotherapy ceased. The rule of thumb seems to be to continue the therapy for two or three years after you begin having few or no symptoms during allergy season.

Put the Brakes on Diabetes

12

*An easy-to-follow action plan
that puts you in the driver's seat.*

Don't be so defensive. Research suggests that most people with diabetes would do well to assume an offensive position. That is, to commit to an aggressive daily action plan designed not just to manage the disease and keep it from getting worse but to actually shift the disease process into reverse.

Imagine requiring less medication to control your blood sugar swings—or perhaps weaning yourself off medication altogether—while preventing the often crippling and deadly complications of diabetes. In fact, not only is this possible but, for people with non-insulin-dependent diabetes (also known as Type II diabetes), the results can be phenomenal.

In one study, 701 people with Type II diabetes—all enrollees at the Pritikin Longevity Center in Santa Monica, California—were asked to follow a challenging diet and exercise regimen. They ate a diet high in complex carbohydrates and fiber and very low in protein and fat. (The therapeutic diet consisted of about 10 percent of calories from fat, compared with the typical American diet of 40 percent fat.) They also walked about 45 minutes each day and participated in a 40- to 50-minute exercise class five times a week.

At the outset, 207 of them were taking oral drugs to control their blood sugar levels. Another 214, who had more advanced cases of diabetes, were on insulin injections. The rest were not on medication of any kind.

After three weeks on the aggressive program, however, 70 percent of the group on oral agents were able to discontinue their medication. Even those whose disease had progressed to the point where they required insulin benefited—36 percent of them were able to go completely medication free. Many in the study were also able to at least reduce their medication requirements.

97

Why Is Insulin So Important?

Your body needs insulin to help turn the foods you eat into energy. Your stomach breaks carbohydrates down into glucose, a common sugar. In response, the pancreas produces insulin, which is needed to take the glucose from the bloodstream into the muscles, where it's either stored or converted to energy.

More than 90 percent of the 14 million people in the United States who have diabetes have Type II. In Type II diabetes, either the pancreas doesn't produce enough insulin to meet the body's needs or the body isn't able to use insulin properly, usually as a result of malfunctioning insulin-receptor cells. (Insulin receptors take up glucose in muscles and other body tissues.)

In people with Type I diabetes, the pancreas produces no insulin at all. People with Type I are dependent on insulin, usually from self-administered injections (although some are turning to new insulin pumps that are surgically implanted under their skin), to keep blood sugar levels normal.

Lifestyle Changes Help Head Off Complications

The implications are clear. An aggressive diet and exercise program can have a major impact on the course of diabetes. And the earlier in the disease process you start making these lifestyle changes, the greater the potential benefits.

"We know that genetic factors predispose certain people to diabetes. But all of the data suggest that lifestyle factors, particularly diet and exercise, can determine whether those genetic factors actually manifest in the disease," says James Barnard, Ph.D., professor of physiological science at the University of California at Los Angeles, an author of the study.

"By committing yourself to certain lifestyle changes, you may be able to reduce your need for medication—and possibly get off and stay off diabetes drugs for the rest of your life," Dr. Barnard continues. "Plus, you may be able to avoid any complications."

The Pritikin program participants saw all three of their heart disease risk factors—total cholesterol, LDL cholesterol and triglycerides—drop dramatically. This is significant because diabetes can double, triple or even quadruple your risk for heart disease. In fact, heart disease is the number-one cause of death among people with diabetes.

"Even Type I diabetics, who must rely on insulin injections, may benefit from a lifestyle approach such as the one described above," Dr. Barnard says. There's a chance that they can reduce the amount of insulin they need to keep their blood sugar levels stable—and that may mean fewer daily injections. And they may also reduce their risk of heart disease and other complications.

Catch It Early

The earlier you take action against diabetes, the better. Unfortunately, the disease is hard to detect at its earliest stages. Here are some things to look for.

■ Check your family tree. Your risk of developing Type I or especially Type II increases if someone in your family is diabetic, particularly if one or both of your parents are.

■ Be alert to the classic symptoms—frequent urination, chronic thirst and increased appetite. If you notice these problems, see a doctor and have your blood sugar tested.

■ Check your scale. Sometimes the only way to know you're insulin resistant—short of a blood test or urine test—is by looking at your bathroom scale. "If you've got a family history of Type II diabetes, being overweight can overburden the system and lead to overt disease," says Marie Gelato, M.D., Ph.D., associate professor of medicine at State University of New York Health Science Center at Stony Brook.

■ Be alert to other warning signs that may accompany classic symptoms. They aren't in themselves reason to believe you have diabetes, but they can help you recognize the presence of the major symptoms. They include weight loss, blurred vision, fatigue, genital or anal itching, yeast infections (in women) and impotence (in men).

■ **Check your blood pressure and lipid levels.** Researchers don't know why, but people with hypertension are more likely to develop diabetes. You're also more susceptible if your total cholesterol is 240 or higher or if your triglycerides are 250 or higher.

Taking Control

Some people with diabetes believe they can simply adjust their medications to compensate for dietary indiscretions. That's their idea of being in control. In fact, says Dr. Gelato, "medications are an adjunct to—not a replacement for—a good diet and exercise program." Real control of diabetes comes from the ability to redirect the course of the disease through a proactive diet and exercise plan coupled with intelligent self-care.

But before you do anything, talk with your doctor. With his or her guidance, you can decide which of these 12 recommended daily actions might best help you achieve your health goals.

1. Monitor Your Blood Sugar Levels throughout the Day ▶ "It's absolutely imprudent to adjust your diet, exercise schedule or medication simply on the basis of the way you feel," says James Pichert, Ph.D., associate professor of education in medicine at the Diabetes Research and Training Center at Vanderbilt University School of Medicine in Nashville, Tennessee.

You can eliminate the guesswork about your diet by using do-it-yourself, at-home blood glucose meters that analyze a sample of your blood (from a pricked finger).

A once-a-day blood sugar test, scheduled at the same time every day, is the absolute minimum. Your doctor may also advise you to check your blood sugar after meals and before and after exercise.

Be sure to log the results of each test in a special

book (available from your doctor or at most drugstores). That allows you and your doctor to analyze the highs and lows and adjust your diet, exercise and medication accordingly, if necessary.

Always be prepared for the unexpected. One goal of an offensive diabetes control program is to aggressively dodge those dangerous dips in blood sugar that so often plague the defensive players. Still, you may not be able to completely avoid these unexpected events. Your best bet is to be prepared. Make sure you replenish your daily stash of easily toted hard candy, boxed raisins or glucose tablets.

2. Keep a Careful Eye on the Fat You Consume ▶ The American Diabetes Association recommends that you limit fat intake to under 30 percent of calories to redirect the course of the disease and prevent complications.

For one thing, fat calories contribute more to excess body weight than calories from any other source. And excess weight contributes to the development of Type II diabetes. Overweight is no small contributor, either. In early stages of Type II diabetes (characterized by a malfunction of the body's insulin-receptor cells), the loss of excess body weight is sometimes sufficient to reverse the degenerative diabetic process and restore function to the receptor cells.

A number of studies also have suggested that overweight people who have diabetes are more likely to have associated risk factors, including high blood pressure, high triglycerides and high cholesterol. These factors in turn can lead to complications like heart disease and kidney damage.

In addition, dietary fat (especially saturated fat) with its artery-clogging, heart-sabotaging abilities, puts an extra burden on people with diabetes, who are already at higher risk for heart disease.

3. Aim for 40 Grams of Fiber from Complex Carbo-hydrates ▶ Fiber-rich complex carbohydrates break down into glucose more gradually and are slowly absorbed into the bloodstream. So, unlike simple sugars, they don't hit your bloodstream all at once, thus preventing a postmeal blood sugar surge. Combined with exercise, they're also a great way to slim down, which is a definite goal for many of those with Type II diabetes.

Among the best sources of complex carbohydrates are starchy foods, like whole-grain breads, pasta and rice, or foods high in water-soluble fiber, like legumes, oats and barley. Studies indicate that these foods digest especially slowly. Water-soluble fiber turns into a gel when it hits your digestive system, increasing the time it takes for the sugar in food to be absorbed by your body.

Although complex carbohydrates are good blood sugar stabilizers, simple carbos, like sugar, boost your blood sugar levels and add to your calorie count. Other sources of simple carbos you should be wary of include alcohol and fruit.

In addition to causing dangerous blood sugar increases, excessive alcohol affects your body's blood sugar control mechanism by limiting the body's ability to respond rapidly if blood sugar drops too low. You're better off abstaining from alcohol completely or limiting it to special occasions only. Never consume more than 3 ounces of distilled liquor, 8 ounces of wine or 24 ounces of beer during a week.

And fructose, the type of sugar in fruit, doesn't raise blood sugar levels as much as refined sugar, so long as you don't consume too much. You should be able (with your doctor's advice) to have about three servings of fruit a day. One serving's equal to half a banana or a small (two inches across) apple.

Shifting the emphasis toward carbohydrates and fiber means moving away from protein—a smart strategy for people with diabetes. Most high-protein foods, including meat, eggs and cheese, are high in fat, especially saturated fat. Plus, "protein puts an extra burden on the kidneys—and kidney disease is a major complication of diabetes," says Monroe Rosenthal, M.D., an endocrinologist and director of the Pritikin Longevity Center. For that reason, it's wise to allow yourself no more than two 3½-ounce pieces of lean meat or fish per day (roughly the size of a deck of cards). Other good sources of protein, such as skim milk and nonfat yogurt, can be eaten in moderation, perhaps two to three cups per day.

4. Take a 45-Minute Exercise Break Every Day ▶
Divide your time between aerobic conditioning and resistance training. "Make exercise just as important and routine as brushing your teeth. Do it every day," Dr. Barnard says. Combined with a low-fat diet, there's no more powerful way to strengthen your resistance to diabetes.

A study of 5,990 men showed that, for every 500 calories burned per week (the equivalent of walking just five miles), the risk of developing Type II diabetes dropped 6 percent.

But the big returns were for the men who had at least one risk factor for the disease, like a family history of diabetes or excess body weight. Men in that high-risk group who burned 2,000 calories or more a week had 41 percent less risk compared with men who burned only 500 calories a week. That's about 45 minutes of brisk walking or stationary cycling.

What's more, research suggests that resistance training may help control blood sugar levels even in those with Type I diabetes. Muscles apparently take up glucose greedily. And there's some evidence that when you build muscle, the muscle's insulin receptors on the cells, which store glucose, may grow in number, and this may enhance glucose utilization by the cells. That means you now have more room to store glucose. With less glucose in circulation, it's possible that insulin requirements may be reduced.

One note of caution: Check with your doctor before beginning any exercise program. And, if your program includes weight training, have your eyes checked regularly. Resistance training may cause surges in blood pressure, which could affect pressure in the eyes.

To reap the benefits of an exercise program, you've got to commit to exercising every day. Here are some tips that may help you make it a daily habit.

■ Schedule your workout the day before, so you establish a routine that's easy to slip into.

■ Lay out your workout clothes for the following day or pack your gym bag every evening.

■ Choose your workout time with regard to your eating schedule. Exercise causes blood sugar levels to drop; if your level slips too far, you may become dizzy, weak and disoriented, a condition known as hypoglycemia. Most experts say the best time to exercise is when your blood sugar level is only slightly elevated. For many people, that's between 60 and 90 minutes after eating.

■ Consider scheduling your workouts in the morning. That's when your energy's most likely to be high, and you're less likely to run the risk of interference.

■ Keep an exercise log in which you note your goals and progress.

5. Consider Supplementing Your Diet ▶ A number of studies suggest that people with diabetes tend to run low on certain vitamins and minerals, particularly vitamins C and E. That's significant because there's increasing evidence that these antioxidant vitamins may offer protection from common diabetes complications, such as heart disease and kidney, eye and nerve damage.

"Because diabetics are prone to vascular disease, they may need to increase their intake of vitamin C," says Ishwarlal Jialal, M.D., assistant professor of internal medicine and clinical nutrition at the University of Texas Southwestern Medical Center in Dallas. He believes people with diabetes should be sure to get 120 milligrams of vitamin C a day—twice the Recommended Dietary Allowance. "That won't cause any side effects, and it could be beneficial," he says.

Vitamin E may prevent a process called protein glycosylation (gleye-caw-sil-A-shun). In a diabetic, this process may be involved in damaging proteins circulating in the blood. By damaging the blood vessels, those renegade proteins may contribute to heart disease and kidney, nerve and eye damage.

Preliminary studies suggest that vitamin E may stop this process from happening. In one small pilot study, for example, researchers gave one group of ten people with Type I diabetes a daily dose of 1,200 milligrams of vitamin E. Another group of ten received 600 milligrams each day, and a third, control group took a look-alike blank pill. After two months, both groups taking vitamin E had significantly lower levels of damaged proteins in their bodies, compared with the control group. And those taking the higher vitamin dose showed better results than those taking the lower-dose pills.

"This study indicates vitamin E may help with the complications so often seen in diabetes," says Stanley Mirsky, M.D., clinical professor of metabolic diseases at Mount Sinai School of Medicine in New York. "We know glycosylation is related to hardening of the arteries and diabetic nerve damage, and we think that might be what makes the kidneys malfunction."

Larger clinical trials are needed to confirm these results. There are also hints that low levels of the minerals chromium and magnesium may also somehow be linked to diabetes.

You can further boost nutrient levels by making smart food choices. Although your fruit servings may be limited (to balance out your meal plan), some vegetables rank high as sources of vitamin C, too. One cup of boiled broccoli is equal to a 116-milligram dose of the heart-healthy vitamin, and an equal amount of brussels sprouts packs a 97-milligram dose. And good, low-fat sources of vitamin E include sweet potatoes, kale, yams and spinach.

6. Consider a Low-Dose Aspirin Daily ▶ New research from the National Institutes of Health (NIH) on 3,711 people with diabetes (either Type I or II) confirms that aspirin can reduce the risk of heart attack and stroke among those with diabetes by as much as 20 percent. "We saw the same reduction in risk in diabetics as other studies have shown with nondiabetics who take aspirin," says Frederick Ferris, M.D., chief of the Clinical Trials Branch at the NIH. "People with diabetes are much more likely to have cardiovascular disease, so the aspirin recommendation is even more relevant for them."

The daily dosage of aspirin used in this study was 650 milligrams, which was much higher than the dose that proved effective in other studies.

"Most researchers agree that the lower dose—equivalent to half an adult aspirin or one children's aspirin—probably has the same effect as the higher dose," Dr. Ferris says. Of course, be sure to talk with your doctor before taking aspirin on a daily basis. Aspirin therapy is ill-advised for people taking blood thinners, for example.

Here's one concern you can put to rest, however: Even if you have diabetic retinopathy, it should be safe for you to take this small dose of aspirin daily. In the above study, the participants taking aspirin were no more likely to experience bleeding from the abnormal blood vessels in the eye than the placebo group.

7. Take Time Out ▶ Preliminary studies suggest that you may be able to control blood sugar levels better if you learn to relax.

In a study at Duke University Medical Center in Durham, North Carolina, doctors first adjusted the diet and medication of 40 people who were having trouble controlling their Type II diabetes. Then the subjects were divided into two groups. One group received intensive diabetes education and participated in progressive relaxation training (in which muscles are tensed and then relaxed, in sequence) twice a week for eight weeks. They also were given relaxation tapes to listen to once a day, or whenever they felt anxious or stressed. The other study group participated only in the diabetes education program.

At 24-week and 48-week follow-ups, the researchers found that, while the relaxation training did not have a significant effect on blood sugar levels in the average patient, it did benefit those under stress. "People who suffered anxiety and complained of stress showed an improvement in blood sugar control when relaxation was added to their regimen," says Richard S. Surwit, Ph.D., professor of medical psychology at Duke and one of the authors of the study.

Hormones like adrenaline, which are activated when you're under considerable stress, are intimately involved in the control of blood sugar. "If your blood sugar drops too low, the brain sends out a signal to increase these stress hormones, and they immediately begin pumping stored glucose into your bloodstream," Dr. Surwit says. "Improving glucose control through stress management may, in theory, prevent some of the complications of diabetes."

Progressive relaxation is only one way to manage stress, of course. Meditation, yoga, guided imagery or a simple walk in the woods may be what works for you.

8. Treat Yourself to a Daily Foot-Care Ritual ▶ Diabetic nerve damage and poor circulation due to high blood sugar levels leave people with diabetes especially vulnerable to skin infections. Your feet, the highest-traffic area on your body, are particularly prone. To prevent these infections—or to nip them in the bud—follow this daily checklist.

■ Shower or bathe in warm (not hot) water. Avoid soaking too long in the tub—it can leave your skin dry and prone to cracks. Be especially careful to dry between your toes to prevent fungal infections.

■ Moisturize. While your skin is still damp after bathing, smooth on a moisturizing lotion. This can help keep the skin on your feet soft and prevent cracks that can open you up to infection.

■ Trim your toenails. To prevent ingrown toenails, make sure that they are carefully clipped straight across and sharp edges are filed with a cardboard nail file.

■ Do a foot inspection. "Look for signs of cracking, peeling and red or irritated skin," says Ellie Strock, R.N., diabetes nurse specialist at the International Diabetes Center. "If you can't see the bottoms of your feet, use a mirror." Blisters, sores, corns, calluses and ingrown toenails should be caught early and treated.

"Weak muscles or shortened tendons due to diabetes-related nerve damage may cause changes in the shape of your feet," she adds. "Be on the alert for those changes—

107
■

they may mean you need to make sure your shoes fit properly and aren't rubbing against the foot, causing pressure."

9. Brush Your Teeth after Every Meal ▶ And floss before bed. Proper dental care is a strategic offensive move that's especially crucial for those with diabetes, because poor blood circulation and possible nerve damage put you at higher risk for infection and gum disease.

10. Drink Eight Eight-Ounce Glasses of Water a Day ▶ Fluid replacement is important for everyone who exercises, but heatstroke, dehydration and the damage they do to the body may be especially dangerous for people with diabetes.

11. Share Time with a Friend ▶ It could be a short phone call or a leisurely lunch. Although all scientific data aren't in yet, some studies do suggest that people with a strong, supportive network of friends and family may be better able to cope with diabetes. Perhaps the roar of the crowd on the sidelines may help keep you motivated to stick to your regimen, and that means you may stay healthier in the long run.

Educating others about the diabetes lifestyle can also help you avoid communication problems. "You need to tell your family and friends exactly what a good diabetic diet is, that you're serious about taking care of yourself and that you'd appreciate their support," says Andrea Anderson, a lifestyle counselor at the Pritikin Longevity Center.

Support groups are also a good way of sharing information and experiences. The American Diabetes Association (703-549-1500), the Juvenile Diabetes Foundation (212-889-7575) and many local hospitals conduct groups and workshops.

12. Reward Yourself ▶ Although you're reaping big bonuses—healthwise—for sticking to your daily schedule, some days it may seem like a lot of effort. Positive reinforcement promotes enthusiasm and motivation to continue with your exercise program. A daily pat on the back is a good way to keep yourself up and motivated. "Take a three-day weekend or get a soothing massage," Anderson suggests. "We're really good at getting down on ourselves when we don't do it right—we need to lift ourselves up and reward ourselves when we do."

One last but important reminder: Check with your physician before changing your routine. New patterns of exercise or diet can alter your metabolism, and you may be told to check in more regularly to see how these changes are affecting you and your need for medication.

Hot Relief 13

This naturally fiery chemical stops pain fast.

We've all done it once or twice in our lives—mistakenly bitten into a hot pepper during a spicy meal. Our mouths turn to fire, and cup after cup of ice water seems only to fan the flames.

Here's the irony—what creates that fiery blast in your mouth may also offer immense relief in certain diabolically painful syndromes.

It's called capsaicin (cap-SAY-i-sin)—the potent fiery extract from hot peppers. In syndromes where pain-transmitting nerves go haywire, causing intense treatment-resisting discomfort, capsaicin may be the spicy switch that turns off the pain and irritation.

Curb Those Nerves

When capsaicin was first fingered as a potent pain fighter, some researchers attributed its magic to so-called counterirritant properties. By creating a burning sensation when rubbed on the skin, capsaicin tricked the brain into focusing on that feeling instead of the other pain or discomfort occurring before. The brain drops what's at hand—it now has other things to worry about.

Now researchers realize capsaicin's power is more than skin deep. Instead of simply acting as an irritating agent on the skin, the extract may reach down further and hit nerve cells that contain something called substance P, which helps transmit pain to and from the brain.

When you first apply capsaicin, substance P is unleashed from nerves leading from the skin, which may cause you to feel some initial burning. After repeated applications, capsaicin keeps these nerves from replenishing their supply of substance P. The nerves run out of their pain-transmitting fuel, so less pain makes it to the brain. Because substance P is the pit bull of pain-transmitting proteins and plays a role in a number of painful syndromes, this simple mechanism of herbal interference may turn out to play a vital, beneficial role in providing substantial relief to many people. Researchers are finding, too, that the pepper-extract rub may work for itching problems as well.

The Pain-Pounding Hit List

Capsaicin (brand names Zostrix and Zostrix HP) has attracted attention mostly for its effects on postherpetic neuralgia and diabetic neuropathy, with preliminary, though encouraging, studies coming out on arthritis. Now, research is making the case even clearer. Here's an update.

Neuropathy ▶ Diabetic neuropathy produces an intense, burning pain that afflicts roughly half of all long-term diabetics, usually staking out their feet. Earlier studies suggested capsaicin can be effective in lessening pain in some of these patients. Now more encouraging research is mounting.

In one study involving 22 neuropathy patients, capsaicin or a placebo cream was applied to painful areas four times a day. Pain measurements were taken at the beginning of the study and at two-week intervals for eight weeks.

Half of those receiving the real cream reported significantly less discomfort—and after four to five months, another 25 percent reported complete cure of the pain. The remaining 25 percent, however, showed no effect from capsaicin. Those getting the placebo cream showed little change in pain. "Nearly all the patients involved had moderate to severe pain that wasn't responding to conventional therapy," says head investigator Rup Tandan, M.D., assistant professor of neurology at the University of Vermont College of Medicine in Burlington. "Here, however, there was definite improvement, especially against burning kinds of pain. It also helped to a lesser degree against stimulus-induced pain—the kind brought on by simply touching the skin with clothes or socks."

"Capsaicin works in about 70 percent of the patients I've tried it on so far," says George Daily, M.D., head of the Division of Diabetes and Endocrinology at Scripps Clinic and Research Foundation in La Jolla, California. "Since it's applied to the skin, you can avoid some side effects associated with the internal drug treatments for diabetic neuropathy like anticonvulsants and antidepressants."

Pruritus ▶ Capsaicin is getting high marks for tackling chronic itching syndromes. For the first time, investigators have pitted capsaicin against a relentless itching, or pruritus, that patients undergoing hemodialysis often experience, with encouraging results. A small group of patients undergoing this blood-purifying process applied a capsaicin cream to problem spots four times daily for six weeks. In this study, eight of nine patients reported significant relief or complete resolution during the study period. In a smaller group, two patients out of five reported complete relief. The spots that received a dummy cream showed much less benefit or none at all.

"It's not known why hemodialysis-related pruritus occurs," says Debra L. Breneman, M.D., of the University of Cincinnati Department of Dermatology. "Regardless of the cause, the itching is often resistant to conventional treatments like antihistamines and steroids,

111

which also carry side effects. Capsaicin, though, may offer an effective alternative with very minor side effects." The initial burning experienced by some patients at the start of their treatments generally lessens in time, she says.

Capsaicin's success once again may boil down to substance P. "We believe that, similar to the way it blocks pain, capsaicin prevents the transmission of the itching sensation from the skin to the brain by depleting substance P from the nerves," says Dr. Breneman.

Because few people receive hemodialysis, studies like this are rare. But Dr. Breneman hopes that capsaicin can be tested in larger groups and compared with other treatments. "Capsaicin may also prove useful in other syndromes where itching is a big problem," she adds.

THE RIGHT WAY TO RUB

"Applying capsaicin cream incorrectly may actually make the pain worse," says Rup Tandan, M.D., a neurologist at the University of Vermont College of Medicine. "That's why it's very important you understand the precautions first and follow instructions fully when using the cream."

Dr. Tandan uses capsaicin primarily with patients experiencing pain from diabetic neuropathy, but his advice should be heeded by anyone using capsaicin cream for other problems as well. Here are his tips on the right way to rub.

• Use a glove or some kind of finger covering when applying the cream. "If you get the cream on your hands and then touch your eyes, it stings like crazy," he says. And don't accidentally touch your nose, lips or eyes with the glove, unless you're prepared to sneeze, cough or cry. "Even though the capsaicin is highly diluted, it's still strong stuff," says Dr. Tandan.

• Take a very small amount of cream and rub it gently over the painful area. When you're finished, there should

Neurodermatitis ▶ This is a chronic itch-and-scratch syndrome, where scratching only incites a more diabolical itch. It's also known as lichen simplex chronicus. "I've used capsaicin on a few patients who scratch themselves crazy, and it seems to work, though research needs to confirm this," says Norman Levine, M.D., professor and chief of dermatology at the Arizona Health Sciences Center in Tucson. "Even though the initial burning is a problem at first, capsaicin may still provide a worthwhile therapy."

Notalgia Paresthetica ▶ This another scratch-like-mad syndrome. It's characterized by an intense itching on a patch of skin on the upper legs, back and shoulder blades. It might be called a meaner, though rarer, cousin of lichen

be a film so fine that you can't see it. "If in between applications you see crusting in the area, you're putting on too much," says Dr. Tandan. The amount you apply may vary. A small dab might do for a finger joint, but a larger amount may be called for by the knee.

• Don't apply the cream within two hours of a hot bath or shower. Heat intensifies the burning caused by the cream and may make the pain you already feel much worse.

• Try out the milder concentration first. The drug comes in two strengths, both of which have been used in various studies. Zostrix is the milder form, with a concentration of 0.025 percent. The stronger form is Zostrix HP, which has three times the power, at 0.075 percent. "Start out with the milder form to see if that does the trick," says Dr. Tandan. If you're already using the higher concentration and you find the burning too much, go back to the milder strength, he says.

• Remember above all that this treatment takes time. In most cases, people respond in a few days to several weeks. Don't be discouraged by the initial burn—you'll need to keep at it to get results.

simplex chronicus. Sufferers have been known to describe the itch as "a crawling sensation" or "a feeling of hot water running down the back, alternating with cold water."

Topical corticosteroids and antihistamines have been used, but again with mixed results. One study, though, looked at case histories of ten patients who reported improvement after applying capsaicin five times daily for one week and then three times daily for three to six weeks. Following treatment, all patients reported milder itching and a reduced frequency of attacks. Some patients relapsed after stopping treatment, but after renewing it, they reported relief. Because these were case reports without placebo comparison, it's not known how much the act of simply rubbing on a cream believed to be effective might have influenced the results.

Neuralgia ▶ We know getting shingles is no day at the beach. But when the blisters finally begin to fade away, pain that lingers for weeks, months or even years can remain as an awful reminder. Doctors call this postherpetic neuralgia (PHN).

Studies have suggested that capsaicin treatment can offer short-term relief for PHN without serious side effects. But scientists haven't been sure that the treatments are safe for long-term use. Now research is answering that question.

In one study, patients with persistent PHN pain were followed as they continued using capsaicin regularly for two years or until they felt no more pain. Capsaicin seemed to offer consistent relief without any major side effects. The burning from the initial application did not build over time, and patients were able to tolerate that unavoidable, initial reaction with little problem.

"We find that as patients get better, we can appropriately cut down the frequency of usage without much problem," says Larry Millikan, M.D., chairman of the Department of Dermatology at Tulane University Medical College in New Orleans. "And in time the patients overcome the burning discomfort they feel when they first use capsaicin. When the relief starts to hit, it really is impressive."

Arthritis ▶ Research has showed that capsaicin cream can help relieve knee pain caused by rheumatoid arthritis and osteoarthritis. Now there is some evidence that capsaicin may help reduce joint pain and tenderness in arthritic fingers, as well.

In one study, capsaicin eased tenderness by 30 percent and pain by 40 percent in the osteoarthritic joints of a group of 21 patients when compared with a placebo cream. In a study of 31 patients, capsaicin was also pitted against pain and tenderness caused by rheumatoid arthritis, and some benefit was shown.

"Capsaicin may be very useful for osteoarthritis of the hands, particularly in people who might have bad reactions to nonsteroidal anti-inflammatory medications," says study author G. M. McCarthy, M.D., assistant professor of medicine in the Division of Rheumatology at the Medical College of Wisconsin in Milwaukee. "Further studies will make it clearer, but capsaicin's role in reducing osteoarthritis pain looks especially good."

On the Capsaicin Frontier

In exciting, newer areas of investigation, capsaicin is just getting its turn at the research bat. Much of this work is fresh and unconfirmed. Keep in mind that these treatments are given in carefully controlled research settings. Don't try capsaicin on your own for these kinds of problems.

Cluster Headaches ▶ Cluster headaches come on like invisible prizefighters, tormenting their victims with recurring bouts of pain concentrated around one eye. Each attack cluster can bring dozens of headaches daily for months and even longer.

In preliminary studies, researchers in Italy targeted cluster headaches with a special nasal spray using capsaicin as its main ingredient.

In one study, 20 adults suffering from long-term and episodic cluster headaches were given a squirt of capsaicin solution in their noses each day for five consecutive days.

The mean number of attacks recorded ten days

115

before treatment was roughly 27. Within ten days of the last application, the number of attacks dropped by about 67 percent. Seven of the 13 patients with episodic cluster headaches experienced complete disappearance of pain attacks after treatment. In three other cases, the number of attacks fell by 75 percent. The number of spontaneously occurring bouts was also greatly reduced even 60 days after the end of treatment.

Since it's tough to make a placebo that can reproduce capsaicin's burning feeling so patients won't know if they're getting the real McCoy or not, this research went without one. Until a successful placebo spray can be found for comparison, results like these should be considered preliminary.

And if the idea of putting something peppery up your nose sounds frightening, it should. Right now there's no commercially available formulation that can be sprayed into that orifice. But the makers of Zostrix are working on it. "Until then we strongly recommend against people using capsaicin cream in nasal passages," says Jean Rumsfield of GenDerm, the makers of Zostrix and Zostrix HP.

Herpes ▶ Right now, herpes research using capsaicin is only in the crawling stages, but the initial findings are intriguing enough to spur wider studies. Research suggests that capsaicin could possibly have some kind of antiviral power—holding the herpes virus hostage so it won't display itself on the skin in the form of fever blisters and lesions.

In one study using herpes-infected guinea pigs, capsaicin treatment didn't prevent disease, but it did make it much less severe compared with untreated animals. These initial data suggest that the virus, which hides in nerve cells between outbreaks, can still move from the skin to the spine but that capsaicin blocks the return trip, preventing the virus from moving to the skin, where it produces the lesions.

"This research is extremely preliminary, though the idea of capsaicin somehow interfering with the way viruses spread is indeed exciting," says Ara H. Der

Marderosian, Ph.D., professor of pharmacognosy and medical chemistry at the Philadelphia College of Pharmacy and Science. "Like the way capsaicin interrupts transmission of pain sensations, it may hinder the transport of virus in the body."

Rhinitis ▶ Rhinitis is a common problem with many symptoms, including nasal blockage, recurrent sneezing and itching. Steroids and antihistamines have been tried with mixed results. Even worse, sufferers can turn their nasal sprays into pint-sized security blankets. Preliminary research, however, suggests that a capsaicin spray may be able to reduce the problems associated with rhinitis while choking off the need for nasal sprays.

One European study targeted 16 adults suffering from severe, chronic, nonallergic rhinitis who had been using nasal sprays for at least a year. They tried the capsaicin spray once weekly for five weeks. Nasal obstruction, runny nose and sneezing frequency were evaluated throughout the study. Following treatment, all symptoms significantly improved during a six-month follow-up period.

In this study, the researchers also looked at the presence of a substance called calcitonin gene-related peptide (CGRP), which is present in the sensory nerves and may play a key role in causing inflammation. They found a 50 percent reduction in the amount of CGRP-like immunoreactivity in nasal biopsies when compared with a control group. Even more, patients were able to be weaned from the other nasal agents after capsaicin treatment.

An earlier study from Italy also showed promising effects using capsaicin against rhinitis. The drug was sprayed into 20 patients' noses three times daily for three days. One month following treatment, both the nasal obstruction and nasal secretion were reduced by roughly 50 percent, while vasoconstrictor nasal spray use during the one-month follow-up period also dropped.

In both studies, patients reported burning discomfort from the spray, which stopped once treatment ended.

117

Especially
for
Women

Your Breast Protection Plan

14

There's a lot you can do to reduce the cancer risk.

You sigh with relief when you find nothing during a breast self-exam. You celebrate every good mammogram report. You feel free from the clutches of worry each time your doctor declares that your breasts are clear of cancer.

Then, after a moment's elation, you cross your fingers and pray your luck continues.

What else can a woman do?

We know that monthly breast self-exams, combined with regular physician exams and mammograms, offer today's best defense against breast cancer. When teamed with state-of-the-art treatment, these measures can help nip cancer before it rages out of control.

But early detection is just one part of an effective cancer-protection plan. Prevention is the other.

Unfortunately, federal funding for research on breast cancer prevention always fell short. However, the National Institutes of Health have launched a $500 million women's-health study to evaluate a variety of preventive measures for heart disease, osteoporosis and, of course, breast cancer. This long-overdue effort will follow 140,000 women over roughly ten years. But can we afford to wait for these results—and other definitive data on the roles dietary fat, fiber, antioxidants, alcohol and body-fat distribution play in breast cancer—before taking action? Many doctors and researchers believe that the evidence to date is compelling enough to support some changes in our dietary habits and lifestyle now.

The Estrogen Connection

"If we halved our fat consumption and doubled our fiber intake, you could predict up to 50 percent less breast cancer in this country," asserts Leonard Cohen,

Ph.D., cell biologist at the American Health Foundation in New York.

The American Cancer Society isn't willing to make such firm predictions yet. But experts there agree that high-fat diets have been linked to breast cancer, as well as cancers of the uterine lining, colon, prostate and pancreas. Most international comparisons show that the countries whose populations consume the most fat, like the United States, have higher breast cancer rates than countries where people eat a very-low-fat diet, like Japan. Scientists looking at the problem on a biochemical level also have reason to believe that fat plays a role in breast cancer.

"One thing we know about breast cancer is that natural estrogens—not the kind that come from birth control pills or estrogen replacement therapy but which are produced naturally in the body—are related to breast cancer risk," says Sherwood Gorbach, M.D., professor of community health and medicine at the Tufts University School of Medicine in Boston.

Dr. Gorbach explains: Women who haven't had children before age 30 face a slightly higher breast cancer risk. That's probably because, without a pregnancy to temporarily diminish estrogen levels, their hormone production continues uninterrupted for years on end. Similarly, women who began menstruating very young or reach menopause very late in life also have slightly higher breast cancer rates, perhaps because their bodies are exposed to estrogen longer.

The encouraging news is that, in tests with 80 women over the past five years, Tufts researchers have found that reducing fats and increasing fiber in the diet causes estrogen levels in the blood to fall.

Fat intake also appears to affect the relative concentrations of estrogen produced in the body. That's what leading researcher Ross Prentice, Ph.D., at the Fred Hutchinson Cancer Research Center in Seattle, has seen in small-scale human studies. "We put 65 post-menopausal women, who had been eating a typical American diet (40 percent of calories from fat), on a low-fat diet (about 20 percent of calories from fat)—in a

120

study initiated by the National Cancer Institute. We found estrogens in the blood decreased within a few weeks." Specifically, levels of blood estradiol, a very active form of estrogen in the body, fell 17 percent.

"We think the implications for breast cancer, as well as endometrial (uterine) cancer, are important," says Dr. Prentice.

The case is far from proved, however. In fact, there are a number of published studies that reject this theory. One of the largest and perhaps most famous studies of its kind, the Harvard Nurses' Study, followed the diets and health of nearly 90,000 nurses for four years. In the end, the researchers found no association between fat intake and breast cancer risk. At least that was the conclusion based on fat-intake levels ranging from 32 to 44 percent of calories.

The Fiber Factor

While the fat debate rages on, scientists are buzzing with new evidence that fiber has the potential to exert even greater breast protection.

Like fat, fiber appears to affect blood estrogen. In one study, scientists from the American Health Foundation examined the effect of dietary fiber on estrogen levels in 62 premenopausal women. The women's daily fiber intake was increased from 15 grams to 30 grams a day, through supplementation with wheat, oat or corn bran.

After two months, the wheat-bran group showed significant reductions in estrogens. The oat and corn bran, however, did not seem to lower estrogen levels.

The same researchers also conducted animal experiments to test fiber's protective power. After exposing animals to a cancer-causing chemical, they found that adding wheat bran to a high-fat diet caused a "highly significant" reduction in breast cancers, compared with animals fed a high-fat, low-fiber diet.

The results of these studies suggest that dietary fiber may reduce breast cancer risk by reducing estrogen levels, the researchers conclude.

In similar studies with small groups of women at

121
∎

Tufts University in Boston, researchers were amazed at the potency of a high-fiber diet. "We were surprised to find that a high-fiber diet plays a more important role than a low-fat diet in reducing (blood) estrogens," notes Dr. Gorbach. "This is a brand-new observation."

He postulates that fiber may bind to the estrogen and carry it from the colon out of the body in the feces.

"The big questions that remain are which fibers and how much," says Dr. Cohen. The safest bet right now is to choose from a wide variety of fiber sources, including whole grains, legumes, fruits and vegetables. The day may come, he says, when better recommendations can be made about the amount and type of fiber people should consume.

Fruits and vegetables are, of course, loaded with fiber. They're also a source of a very special family of vitamins called antioxidants, which may prove to be our secret weapon against breast cancer. A growing number of studies link fruit and vegetable intake or intake of the associated antioxidants—beta-carotene (which converts into vitamin A in the body) and vitamin C—with reduced breast cancer rates. "Up until now breast cancer debates have focused on fat," says Gladys Block, Ph.D., professor of nutrition at the school of public health at the University of California in Berkeley. "I think more people are going to start considering fruits and vegetables for preventing breast cancer."

Researchers at the State University of New York at Buffalo, for example, published a study of 439 postmenopausal breast cancer patients, compared with other age-matched, randomly selected residents of their communities. Women from both groups were interviewed over a two-hour period about their diets.

The scientists found that breast cancer patients consumed fewer nutrient-packed foods like tomato juice, vegetable juice, tomatoes, corn, asparagus, strawberries, apples, grapefruit, lemons and limes. Translating foods into nutrients, the cancer patients consumed less fiber and folate as well as less vitamins E, C and beta-carotene—the so-called antioxidants.

"It's possible that it's the antioxidants that really

work and may reduce the risk of breast cancer," says Saxon Graham, Ph.D., who led the western New York study. The antioxidants trap free radicals, wayward molecules that would otherwise cause many kinds of damage in the body, including damage to DNA molecules that may cause normal cells to go awry.

An analysis of data from the Harvard Nurses' Study backs up the antioxidant hypothesis. The researchers compared 1,439 women who had invasive breast cancer with a group of healthy women. All completed a food-frequency questionnaire in 1980. Eight years later, the researchers found, consumption of vitamin A was related to reduced breast cancer risk. High vitamin E intake was also associated with low risk.

Charles Hennekens, M.D., Dr.P.H., acting head of the Preventive Medicine Department at Harvard Medical School and a collaborator on the nurses' study, says that while these results are interesting, they're not definitive. He points out that the women who ate diets high in antioxidants might also have had other healthy dietary or lifestyle habits. "We will be able to provide reliable information in the future as to whether these micronutrients really prevent cancer or whether they're merely a marker for some other dietary or lifestyle factor," says Dr. Hennekens.

A Word about Crucifers

Before leaving the produce bin, let's take a look at crucifers. Research suggests that increased consumption of these vegetables (including broccoflower, broccoli, brussels sprouts, cabbage, cauliflower, kale and kohlrabi) is associated with lower rates for a variety of cancers.

A unique family of vegetables, crucifers contain a specific class of compounds called indoles. In an animal study at the Institute for Hormone Research in New York City, scientists H. Leon Bradlow, Ph.D., and Jon Michnovicz, M.D., Ph.D., discovered that the indoles may alter estrogen metabolism and so reduce breast cancer risk. The indoles may also block cancer-causing chemicals, according to the researchers.

123
∎

They've demonstrated that one type of indole, called indole-3-carbinol, can reduce breast tumors in animals. And they've begun looking into the effect in humans. In one small study, the scientists administered indole-3-carbinol daily to a dozen people aged 22 to 48. The daily dose was equivalent to the amount you'd get from eating about a pound of raw cabbage or brussels sprouts.

The test lasted seven days, during which the subjects' estrogen metabolism was studied. The scientists found that the subjects experienced an increase in a weak kind of estrogen that's considered less likely to stimulate tumor growth and a decrease in a more active and cancer-promoting form of estrogen. "Their work is very interesting and valuable," comments Christopher Longcope, M.D., breast cancer researcher at the University of Massachusetts in Amherst. "Whether this finding will provide a way to protect against breast cancer requires more research."

"Pear" Down Your Risk

You may believe that eating pears and apples can influence your risk of breast cancer. But would you believe that looking like a pear or an apple can, too? It has to do with body-fat distribution. People who are apple shaped are broad in the middle. Their weight is distributed on the so-called upper-body locations: abdomen, chest, arms and back. Pears, like their namesakes, carry their weight down low, around the buttocks and thighs.

To prevent heart disease, researchers have found that the pear shape is healthier. And now they're drawing a similar conclusion about breast cancer. New evidence is pointing to the likelihood that the location of fat is as important as, or even more important than, the amount of fat when it comes to breast cancer risk.

In one study, Rachel Ballard-Barbash, M.D., of the National Cancer Institute's Division of Cancer Prevention and Control in Rockville, Maryland, examined data on body-fat distribution and breast cancer from some 2,000 women who took part in the Framingham Heart

124

Study (a study of a Massachusetts community aimed primarily at gathering information on risk factors for heart disease). Over 28 years, 106 of the women developed breast cancer.

Dr. Ballard-Barbash found that women with more upper-body fat had a 70 to 100 percent greater risk of developing breast cancer than women whose fat was on their lower body. The association seemed strongest for women past menopause. Measurements of general fatness were not associated with breast cancer risk among these women.

Why might the location of the fat make a difference? Unfortunately, scientists say, fat doesn't just sit there. Body fat, depending on the location, can alter hormonal patterns or be a marker of hormonal metabolism.

Specifically, researchers believe that the location of fat in the body influences estrogen production and metabolism. David Schapira, M.D., chief of cancer prevention at the H. Lee Moffitt Cancer Center and Research Institute and professor of medicine at the University of South Florida College of Medicine in Tampa, first noticed the link between body shape and cancer risk. Apple-shaped women, notes Dr. Schapira, have lower levels of a protein called sex-hormone-binding globulin (SHBG). SHBG binds to estrogen, preventing it from roaming free to act on the breast and other vulnerable tissue (like the uterine lining).

Researchers have observed that breast cancer patients do indeed have lower levels of SHBG, says Dr. Schapira. "These lower levels of SHBG appear to be an important factor in increasing breast and endometrial cancer risk in apple-shaped women."

How can you tell if you're an apple or a pear? Put a tape measure around your waist (at belly-button level). Then measure around your hips, at their widest point. Divide the waist measurement by the hip measurement. (If your waist is 24 inches and your hips 36, for example, your waist/hip ratio is 0.66.) According to Dr. Schapira's research, the lowest risk is incurred by women whose ratio is less than 0.73. If the ratio is higher than 0.75, you're an "apple" and at higher risk for breast cancer.

But don't panic: Body shape is not a life (or death) sentence. It's easier than you might expect to transform an apple into a pear. That's because when fat comes off, it's most likely to disappear from the abdomen, says Dr. Schapira. That's what he found in a study of 124 women in a weight-loss program. Sixty-four percent of the women who lost ten or more pounds effectively reshaped themselves into pears. He estimates that the women who lost ten or more pounds reduced their breast cancer risk by 45 percent.

Whether obesity alone is a risk factor for breast cancer is not known. But most researchers say it's better to be slim than sorry. "I don't think it's particularly good to be overweight, for many reasons," says Dr. Schapira. "Overweight people are probably eating a high-fat, high-calorie diet, and there's fairly good evidence that behavior is linked to breast cancer."

15 Fooling Mother Nature

Easy techniques for concealing small complexion flaws.

It's one of nature's little ironies. You may be fit and feel great. Yet under-eye circles make you look like you're burning the candle at both ends and in the middle.

What to do? If you think you can't fool Mother Nature, read on to discover how cosmetic concealers can help you hide complexion flaws.

Today's concealers come in a wide range of applicators, consistencies and shades. How you choose and apply them can make the difference between erasing a flaw and drawing attention to it. To take the guesswork out of choosing and using concealer, a leading makeup artist shares his techniques and tips for perfect camouflage.

Choose Your Weapon

Your major considerations in choosing the perfect concealer are consistency and color.

"Test a concealer on the area where you're going to be using it before you buy it," says Leonard Engelman, noted Hollywood makeup artist and president of TAUT cosmetics. "The consistency should allow it to go on smoothly and be easy for you to work with. The best concealer will be pigment-dense (to give you maximum coverage) with a consistency that spreads easily for a thin coverage without a 'crepey'-look buildup."

Choosing the best color to hide skin discoloration or bags is relatively easy. A concealer should have the same undertone as your skin and be just a bit lighter. "Your goal in both foundation and concealer is to look natural," says Engelman. "Go with a color that's as close as possible to your own skin tone."

The Art of Coloration

To begin, apply your moisturizer. Now put on the foundation. By doing this you see where you need to apply concealer and avoid using too much.

"I use a sponge for the foundation and then, when it comes to the concealer, I recommend using a small, flat artist's brush. Use short, feathery strokes. A brush lets you apply the concealer to the exact areas you want it," Engelman says.

Where to put your concealer depends on the problem you want to correct. If you want to cover discoloration underneath your eyes (circles), apply it only where the darkness is and blend it into your foundation.

Also check the area between the bridge of your nose and the inner corner of your eye for shadows. "That's a great place to use a concealer and one people often miss," says Engelman. "It helps to enliven the eye, first because you're getting rid of the discoloration and second, when you do your eye makeup you determine the highlights and shadows—the discoloration doesn't determine them."

Another way to think of a concealer is as a highlight.

127

"For a woman with fullness under her eyes, don't bring the concealer over the top of the bag, because that draws attention to the puffiness," Engelman says. What you want to do is to apply the concealer just underneath the puffy area, at the shadow of the bag. So what you're going to do is literally replace shadow with light. In that way you're going to balance out the eye.

If your bags are pronounced, the shadow goes from the bridge of the nose to the outside of the eye. Use the shadow as your guide to determine where to apply your under-eye concealer.

The final step in applying a concealer is to use powder, which absorbs the oil or the moisture in makeup and sets it. Use a fine-milled powder—some brands make their own meant specially to be used with a concealer—but any fine-textured translucent or transparent powder should work well.

"If you have a few lines under your eyes, there's a technique to using powder without it creasing. Just before you powder, make sure you smooth out the area underneath the eye. Then look upward and powder that area," Engelman says. A light film is all you need to do the job.

Flaw-Free Skin

There are other flaws that concealers can help you hide. Pimples call for a somewhat different technique, because you want the concealer, as it hides, to help aid the healing, not exacerbate the problem.

If this type of blemish is a serious problem for you, consult your dermatologist. If it's a once-in-awhile annoyance, you can do it yourself.

There are two ways to approach this problem. One is to use a medicated concealer. The drawback here is that you don't have the range of colors to choose from, and the medicated products are too drying for some sensitive skins.

The other approach is to treat a pimple as a flaw that has to be handled with care. Apply a therapeutic lotion or gel to the blemish so your skin doesn't absorb any oil in the concealer. Be sure that any moisturizer you use around the blemish is either oil free or very lightweight. Be particularly gentle when you apply your concealer. Use either a makeup brush or a sponge, or your ring finger.

Concealers can also hide dark pigmentation elsewhere on your face, such as above the lip line.

"Very few women don't have that," says Engelman. Use a very thin application of concealer. "Apply the major amount of product in the center of the discoloration and just blend it out. As with under-eye circles, apply your concealer over your foundation."

Another use for your concealer is to deemphasize expression lines by using it as a highlighter. This technique works well to soften laugh and frown lines by replacing shadow with light. This can also be done at the corners of the mouth to help lift them.

And there's one little area of the eye that's important to take care of. Where the eyelids come together, at the outer part of the eye, there's usually a little line. That line always goes down because it's going in the direction of the upper lid. "You don't ever want anything leading downward on your face. It ages you. You want to be sure to erase that little line so the eye can go in an upward motion. It's one little thing, but it can make an enormous difference on the eye."

Any woman over 25 knows that her face isn't the only place that can use camouflaging. To conceal scars, age spots, birthmarks and broken blood vessels, give them the same treatment as under-eye circles. Naturally you also powder these when you're done, to set the makeup.

Companies that actually specialize in corrective cosmetics for the face, such as Covermark and Dermablend, also make excellent waterproof products specially formulated to help hide unsightly veins on the legs. These also work well on the hands or arms.

A Health Bonus

It's unusual to talk about a genuine health bonus from cosmetic regimens, but for concealers it's possible. Because the pigment in them is dense, concealers offer an automatic additional sunscreen for the delicate under-eye area and help stop further hyperpigmentation (or age spots) caused by the sun.

This doesn't mean you don't need a sunscreen, but a concealer does give you an added degree of protection. In fact, some companies have added sunscreens to their concealers.

16   Is "Feminine Hygiene" Worthwhile?

This is one ritual most women can do without.

David A. Eschenbach, M.D., has one carefully considered word for the estimated one-third of American women who douche regularly—"Don't."

Dr. Eschenbach, a professor of obstetrics and gynecology at the University of Washington in Seattle, has coauthored a study that linked douching to pelvic inflammatory disease (PID), a potentially serious bacterial infection of the uterus, fallopian tubes and ovaries. PID causes severe lower abdominal pain and threatens fertility.

The study does not prove that douching *causes* PID, but it confirms an association women's health experts have suspected for many years.

"Douching reminds me of smoking," Dr. Eschenbach says. "Women spend an estimated $100 million a year on douches. The practice has no known health benefits. And it's associated with significant health risks, not just PID but also vaginal infections and ectopic (tubal) pregnancy, which can cause life-threatening complications."

The four-year study involved almost 1,000 women aged 16 to 50, treated at Harborview Medical Center in Seattle—100 with confirmed PID, 119 with lower abdominal pain that turned out not to be PID and 762 in a control group who sought treatment for other reasons.

In exhaustive two-hour interviews, researchers asked them hundreds of standardized questions about their medical histories and lifestyles. Compared with those who douched less than once a month, the women who douched three or more times a month had 3.6 *times* the risk of developing PID.

A Dangerous Practice

"We have two theories why women who douche might be at increased risk for PID," Dr. Eschenbach says. "The physical action of douching may push PID-causing microorganisms from the vagina up into the uterus. Or douching might change the chemical environment of the vagina so that more of these organisms grow there, and then some of them might work their way up into the reproductive organs. It's also possible that both factors are at work."

No particular type of douche was more strongly associated with PID. Commercial douches and homemade vinegar-and-water solutions both increased the risk of pelvic infection. "We found a slight tendency for commercial douches to be riskier," Dr. Eschenbach explains, "but it wasn't statistically significant."

Nonetheless, he says he's "personally more concerned" about commercial douches. "The more ingredients a douche contains, the greater the risk that one or more of them can cause harm. The commercial products contain perfumes, preservatives, and chemicals like the disinfectant phenol, things I consider causes for concern."

Gynecologists have suspected a link between douching and pelvic inflammatory disease for almost 40 years. A study published in 1985 linked douching to an increased risk of ectopic pregnancy, fetal development in a fallopian tube instead of the uterus. Physicians consider ectopic pregnancy a medical emergency because as the fetus grows, the fallopian tube eventually ruptures, causing bleeding and potentially life-threatening complications. Once diagnosed, usually because of lower abdominal pain on just one side, ectopic pregnancies are terminated surgically.

"We've known for many years that ectopic pregnancy is associated with a history of PID," Dr. Eschenbach says, "so when the study appeared linking ectopic pregnancy to douching, it was only a short step to suspect that douching might be directly linked with PID."

Surprisingly, the women at greatest risk for douching-associated PID were the ones with the *lowest* number of lifetime sexual partners (ten or fewer). "At first glance, this seems odd," Dr. Eschenbach says.

"Usually the more partners a woman has, the greater her risk of reproductive infections. That's certainly the case with gonorrhea and chlamydia. But gonorrhea and chlamydia are independently associated with PID. Women with these sexually transmitted diseases (STDs) have a 10 to 20 percent annual risk of PID even if they don't douche. On the other hand, women with no history of these STDs have a PID risk of less than 1 percent. Douching increases PID risk for all women, but it increases it *a lot more* for women with no STD history, the women with only a few lifetime sexual partners."

Unnecessary Risks

"It's never been clear to me why women douche," says Elena Gates, M.D., an assistant professor of obstetrics and gynecology at the University of California's San Francisco Medical Center. "For many, it seems their mothers taught them it was a regular part of personal hygiene. And for the last 15 years or so, that message has been reinforced by heavy advertising by the makers of commercial douches. I've had many patients express surprise when I informed them douching wasn't necessary."

Douching is unnecessary because the vagina is a self-cleansing organ. "The normal, healthy vagina has effective mechanisms to get rid of dead cells and bacteria," Dr. Gates says. "Occasionally, if a woman has a bad vaginitis, douching might help restore the normal vaginal environment, but routine douching kills off the good *Lactobacillus* bacteria that normally populate the vagina, and it increases risk of vaginal infection as well as PID."

Instead of douching, women interested in improving their vaginal health should wear cotton panties and panty hose with a breathable cotton panel, and wipe from front to back to prevent introducing bacteria from the anal area into the vagina.

They might also try eating yogurt containing live *Lactobacillus acidophilus* bacteria. In a study at Long Island Jewish Medical Center in New York, researcher Eileen Hilton, M.D., showed that one cup of bacteria-rich yogurt a day reduced yeast vaginitis risk by two-thirds. Unfortunately, few yogurts contain live *Lactobacillus*, but Columbo's, distributed in the East, is one brand that does, Dr. Hilton says.

Staying
Fit

Turn Back the Clock

17

An antiaging plan to help you stay strong, work harder and look better.

The exercise revolution is turning the concept of aging—not to mention government policy—on its ear. To decide whether public-safety workers in their sixties are as competent as their younger counterparts, the U.S. government commissioned studies looking at aging's effects on mental and physical ability. Dozens of fire and police departments across the country were targeted for research. Investigators also analyzed reams of studies done on aging to see if more gray hair means less competence.

This notion, which many believe, fell flat on its face. "In fact, we found that many older adults were more fit than other employees years younger than them," says Frank J. Landy, Ph.D., from the Center for Applied Behavioral Sciences at Pennsylvania State University in University Park. "Aging did not play a key role—physical and mental fitness dictated their effectiveness."

The occupations under study were firefighter, prison guard and police officer—jobs where quickness, strength, vitality and overall health really matter. Yet, if a police officer cannot operate effectively, it's not because he's 57 instead of 27. It's because he's let himself go—with too many evenings in front of the TV and too many breakfasts at the doughnut counter.

This exciting research suggests that fitness in many ways makes aging irrelevant. Birthdays are simply arbitrary signposts on a highway—telling you how far you've gone but having little bearing on the quality of the journey ahead.

The real marker is the human body and its components—bones, muscle, metabolism and cardiovascular system. The better condition they're in, the less likely age can prey on them. Even more, research is making it clearer each day that exercise is the one powerful tool to protect and improve those markers.

Breaking the Age Barrier

We know that exercise—both aerobic and strength training—can make us look and feel years younger, literally from the inside out. All that decays with aging can be reversed with muscle, sweat and a healthy dose of enthusiasm. Among the areas most vulnerable to the functional decline that exercise helps to protect are:

■ Muscle. It withers at a rapid pace in sedentary people as they start to get older.

■ Bone. It may thin with age and inactivity, leading to osteoporosis.

■ Metabolism. It slows as body composition shifts to less muscle and more flab.

■ Joints. Inactivity restricts motion and excess weight causes strain, especially when surrounding muscles are weak.

Even more, research is showing how potent exercise is in reducing risk for strokes and cancer later in life. Add to that the more immediate benefits of lower blood pressure, healthier cholesterol levels and improved management of blood sugar levels, and you have the strongest case yet for establishing a healthy sweat.

And then, of course, there's the obvious: a shapelier, slimmer, firmer figure.

Take Back the Battleground

The exercises prescribed to break the age barrier target those areas especially vulnerable to the constant harassment of Father Time. We're talking about the rusty spots that are the first to go as we gray—gremlins that start to creak, groan and ache in one collective bodily whine. The goal of this program is to polish, buff and oil those shaky and stiff places, bolstering existing weaknesses and preventing others from arising. The battlefronts we have in mind are:

Posture ▶ While eyeing the crow's-feet in the mirror, step back a few feet—you may find an even more obvious sign of advancing years. Posture, or lack of it, can be the mark of successful—or disastrous—aging. As your back slouches, your neck droops and your shoulders fold inward, the little crinkles by the eyelids become insignificant. What's worse, what's going on outside your body is hurting your insides, too.

"As the neck begins to come forward and the back starts to slouch more and more, you actually start cramping up the internal organs," says national YMCA strength consultant Wayne Westcott, Ph.D. "This can get so bad your last rib can actually touch your pelvic girdle." A proper strength-training program, however, can prevent your body from looking like a ? and more like a !. "Posture is a function of muscular strength," says Dr. Westcott. "Exercises that build up and preserve muscles in the neck and back are extremely important in helping to maintain correct posture throughout our lives."

Flexibility ▶ As posture falters with age, so does flexibility, especially in the area of spinal mobility. Rigidity and stiffness can start in our thirties and really speed up in the later decades. Research suggests, however, that adults with restricted mobility can reverse this decline with a simple program using flexibility exercises.

"Strength and flexibility go hand in hand—loss of strength leads to increased stiffness, and thus mobility suffers," says Daniel Kosich, Ph.D., senior director of IDEA, an organization of fitness professionals. By performing exercises that use the entire range of motion of joint and muscle, you enhance flexibility, which has another benefit. "The more flexible you are, the lower your risk for becoming injured," says Dr. Kosich. The strengthening exercises in our ten-point plan also help enhance flexibility.

137

Lean Body Mass ▶ As you age, you can lose about ½ pound of muscle per year. While you lose that, you're loading up on body fat. In fact, between 20 and 80, body fat can jump from 15 to 40 percent in men and from 20 to 40 percent in women.

Think about what that does to your body: You get weaker—while you're carrying more excess baggage around. Plus, that change in body composition wreaks havoc on your metabolism. With less high-metabolism muscle, you burn fewer calories, which means you'll gain even more weight—with much more dreadful ease.

The only way you can prevent this is to preserve and build lean muscle mass. That means strength training—making muscles bigger—which means creating more tissue that's hungrier for calories.

"In one of my studies, people who added strength training to their fitness regimen lost six pounds of fat while actually adding three pounds of muscle mass," says Dr. Westcott.

In the workouts, Dr. Westcott's subjects performed 20 minutes of strength training plus 20 minutes of aerobic exercise three days a week for eight weeks—that's all.

"These people did not diet," says Dr. Westcott. "Strength training improves metabolism with that positive change in body composition, so dieting becomes less important in maintaining healthy body weight and a shapely figure."

The Shoulders ▶ The key shoulder muscles—called rotator-cuff muscles—are often the most neglected muscles on the body when it comes to strengthening exercise, creating an imbalance between the often-used large muscles of the chest and these more obscure muscles.

"It's these small, vulnerable muscles that help maintain the integrity of the shoulder, holding it in good posture," says Dr. Kosich. "Often people with weak rotator-cuff muscles can risk tearing one of them if they engage in any out-of-the-ordinary athletic endeavor, like a weekend softball or volleyball game."

The rolled shoulder—when your upper body hunches

inward, with your chest sinking in—can be tied to weakness and imbalance in muscles of the shoulder girdle. "Some of these muscles really don't get challenged much over a lifetime," says Dr. Kosich. "One common muscle imbalance is directed toward the anterior muscles—the chest muscles—which tend to be stronger than the muscles of the back." To bring a balance into your body, we've included one exercise that targets the shoulder area.

Achieving upper-body balance doesn't mean neglecting the chest muscles, however. One of the largest sets of muscles, the pectoral muscles, are the workhorses of the upper body, called upon in just about any activity requiring upper-body strength. Surveys have shown—frighteningly—that after the age of 74, nearly two-thirds of women cannot lift objects weighing more than ten pounds. Thankfully, a few minutes with light barbells can reverse that decline. By pumping the chest muscles and the upper arm's biceps muscles regularly, you can make sure you end up on the stronger side of the next survey.

The Knee ▶ This joint can wear away to half its strength in just two decades. But this decay may be slowed by building up the muscles around the knee, primarily the quadriceps, hamstrings and, to a lesser extent, the calves.

Strong quadriceps muscles offer more than knee support. "Throughout our lives they're responsible for our movement—when we're going up and down stairs, walking and running," says Dr. Westcott. "By neglecting them, a person is forfeiting the freedom to lead an active life." In fact, the quadriceps muscles can lose 40 to 50 percent of their strength between the ages of 20 and 60 if those years are spent largely inactive. This loss can potentially be reversed, however, by inducting those muscles into a strength-training program.

And if you're going to work the "quads," you have to hit the "hams"—the hamstring muscles located on the back of the thigh. Exercising both groups helps maintain a muscular balance, protecting against extra stress on the knee.

Targeting the calves also helps add some muscular

139

stability to the leg while helping to protect against recurring injuries like shin splints—the aches and pains that occur around the tibia, the bones that make up the shin.

The Skeleton ▸ Women can lose up to 4 percent of bone each year after menopause, which increases the risk for fracture in areas like the spine, forearm and hip. Even worse, half of all falls that involve fractures require hospital admission, with the person discharged to a nursing home.

"By increasing bone density, however, the tendency for calcium leeching to occur from the skeleton is likely reduced," says Dr. Kosich. "Exercise may stimulate the chemistry associated with maintenance and increase of bone." The bolstered bone may in turn reduce fracture risk, throwing a roadblock in the path to the nursing home. In fact, a study showed that among a group of 13,000 older adults, those who actively exercised one or more hours a day had 50 percent less chance of getting a hip fracture than those who didn't exercise.

The Midsection ▸ To really trim fat on the belly, you need a potent stew of aerobic exercise, abdominal work and a healthy, low-fat diet. The benefits aren't just cosmetic. Excess fat around the midsection has been implicated in raising the risk of breast cancer, heart disease and diabetes.

One important component of that strategy—building the abdominal muscles—has other benefits as well. It helps your lower back, a prime target of pain as we get older. Researchers have found a strong correlation between weak stomach muscles and chronic back pain, and that persistent pain may be helped with simple and slow concentrated exercises hitting the abdominal muscles.

The Brain ▸ Humans still have all the markings of hunter-gatherers—creatures who need strenuous activity to survive. It's the emergence of the sedentary lifestyle—sofa, television, remote control and corn chips included—that has softened us, contributing to the deterioration of physiological and cognitive function during so-called normal aging. Here's the good news: Exercise may not only cut risk of physical disease, it also help that mighty "muscle" above the neck that keeps us on our toes. We're talking brain power.

One study, which looked at the effect of age and fitness on various measures of cognition and visual sensitivity in 60 men, offers some encouraging evidence. Researchers found that fitness was associated with better brain performance regardless of age. Scores of the 50- to 62-year-old highly fit men were no different than those of highly fit and less fit young men.

Somehow aerobic fitness confers some level of immunity against functional loss that typically occurs with normal aging. Researchers aren't positive, but they suggest exercise may tune a more efficient central nervous system. We also know working out may make oxygen more available for brain activity. Oxygen is essential for the metabolism of glucose, which maintains brain energy levels, and also for the metabolism of several other brain chemicals like neurotransmitters. Enhanced cognitive function may be due to an even simpler mechanism, however. "Exercise makes you feel better and elevates your confidence," says Dr. Kosich. "That allows you to focus better on the activities at hand, so your work capacity undoubtedly improves."

Exercises That Slow Aging

This antiaging exercise plan focuses on the parts of the body most vulnerable to the aging process. Of course, aerobic exercise is just as important as these body-building weapons. By doing both aerobics and strength training, while eating a low-fat diet, you have a perfect combination to slim down and shape up.

Include one aerobic workout of 30 to 45 minutes at least three to five times a week. Do this with a brisk walk, a healthy jog or an aerobics class of your choice. Perform the exercises below three times a week, with one to three sets of each exercise. Shoot for 8 to 12 repetitions per exercise. When weights or machines are used, always begin with a low, comfortable level of resistance.

141

Increase the resistance slowly over time, and never to the point where you are straining or feeling any discomfort. If you're out of shape or have a medical problem of any kind, get specific clearance from your physician before beginning any exercise program.

Abdominal Curl ▶ This targets back pain, potbelly and abdominal muscles.

Lie on your back with your knees bent and your fingers lightly touching your ears. You can place your hands behind your head as long as you don't use them to pull your head forward. Slowly curl your upper torso only until your shoulders leave the floor. Hold for a few seconds, go down and repeat, inhaling as you go down. If this is too difficult, keep your arms at your sides.

Bench Press ▶ This targets upper-body strength and posture.

Lie on an exercise bench with your knees bent so your feet are flat on the floor. Grasp dumbbells or a barbell (if you're using a barbell, be sure to have a partner to spot you) with your hands slightly more than shoulder-width apart. Slowly lower them to your chest. Press the dumbbells up until your arms are fully extended, with your elbows almost locked. Repeat.

Arm Curl ▶ This targets osteoporosis (forearm) and biceps strength.

Hold the barbell with both hands, palms up. Stand with your back straight, with the bar at arm's length against your upper thighs. Curl the bar up in a semicircular motion until your forearm touches your biceps. Keep your upper arms close to your sides. Lower the bar slowly to the starting position, using the same path.

Seated Quadriceps Extension ▶ This targets mobility, knee stability and padding.

Sit in a "leg machine" with your feet under the pads. Straighten one knee out, then lower your foot back down. Do eight to ten times. Then switch to the other leg. (Use ankle weights if you don't have a machine.)

Bent-Over Dumbbell Row ▶ This targets posture, back flexibility and osteoporosis.

Put your feet close together and place the dumbbells on the floor outside of each foot. Bend forward and grasp the dumbbells. Keep your knees slightly bent and your torso parallel to the floor. Pull the dumbbells straight up to the sides of your chest. Keep your head up and your back straight, and don't let the weights touch the floor.

Seated Barbell Calf Raise ▶ This targets shin splints, knee stability and calf strength.

Place a raised object on the floor about 12 inches away from the end of a bench. Sit at the end of bench. Hold a barbell on your upper thighs (use a pad) about three inches above your knees. Place the balls of your feet on object and raise up on your toes as high as possible. Hold this position momentarily, then return slowly to the starting position.

Neck Exercise ▶ This targets posture.

Sit on a bench with your back straight and your head up. Place both hands on your forehead and push your head back as far as is comfortable while resisting with your neck muscles. Use only moderate resistance. At the low position, push your head back up in a semicircular motion as far as is comfortable. Resist with your neck muscles. Do ten repetitions, then place your hands on the back of your head and repeat the movement in reverse.

Seated Side Lateral Raise ▶ This targets upper-body strength and posture and provides rotator-cuff protection.

Sit on the end of a bench with your feet firmly on the floor. Hold the dumbbells with your palms in and your arms straight down at sides. Raise the dumbbells in a semicircular motion a little above shoulder height. Pause for a moment, then lower to the starting position, using the same path. Keep your arms slightly bent.

143

Hamstring Curl (with Partner) ▶ This targets knee protection, mobility and muscle balance.

Lie face down on a "leg machine," holding on to the front of the machine. Curl your legs up until your calves touch the upper part of your thighs. Return to the down position and repeat. If you don't have a machine, a partner can provide resistance.

Hip Flexer ▶ This targets osteoporosis (hip bone).

Place an ankle strap (or weight) on your left ankle. If you want, you can hold on to a waist-high object in front of you for balance. Keeping your leg straight, with the knee slightly bent, raise your left leg until your thigh is parallel to the floor. Return to the starting position. Keep your back straight throughout the exercise.

18   Eating Smart

It's easy to lose weight without starving yourself—if you make the right choices.

By now, Dean Ornish, M.D., is used to hearing about miracles. He's helped them happen. Ever since he published his landmark research showing that you can reverse heart disease with lifestyle changes alone—no drugs or surgery—he's heard from thousands of people who adopted his program and report amazing results. Many say their cholesterol levels plummeted and their excess weight melted away. Yet they never went hungry; indeed they ate as much and as often as they wanted.

Dr. Ornish isn't a diet doctor; he's an assistant clinical professor of medicine at the University of California and director of the Preventive Medicine Research Institute in Sausalito. But he unexpectedly picked up a lot of insight into the mechanics of weight loss during his research with heart patients. You're probably already aware of the success Dr. Ornish had actually reversing

144
■

patients' heart disease with a lifestyle program that includes a mostly vegetarian regimen with no more than 10 percent of its calories from fat.

In addition to adopting this eating plan, Dr. Ornish's patients made some fairly simple lifestyle changes. They learned how to manage stress, and they took up an exercise program—20 to 60 minutes of moderate exertion, such as walking, at least five times a week.

All of that did more than improve the people's cardiovascular health: It helped them to shed unwanted pounds—an impressive 22 pounds on average over the first year. Without even trying!

And the best part? These folks ate more food, more often, than they did before they started his lifestyle program. Imagine: They weren't hungry; they weren't deprived; they became healthier; and they lost weight! It all sounds too good to be true. But it isn't.

No Calculator Required

"Most 'diets' fail because they're based on deprivation. Cutting calories, restricting portion sizes and reducing the amount of food you eat—that all leaves you feeling hungry. And nobody wants to feel hungry all the time," says Dr. Ornish.

In order to lose weight, he maintains, you need to think about changing the type of food you consume rather than limiting the amount. Just focus your diet on foods that are very low in fat, high in complex carbohydrates and high in fiber. For the most part, vegetarian fare fits the bill—that is, fruits, vegetables, grains and legumes (beans, peas and lentils).

Beyond natural vegetarian fare, Dr. Ornish's eating plan allows nonfat dairy products and nonfat or very-low-fat (and sugar-free or low-sugar) commercial products. That's it.

No meat, poultry, fish, cheese or other high-fat foods are allowed. It's not that it's necessary to eliminate these foods completely in order to maintain a healthy diet with 10 precent of calories from fat. But Dr. Ornish believes that, in some ways, it's easier to eliminate these foods entirely than to cut back on them. "Your palate never gets a chance to readjust if you keep eating meat, even in smaller quantities, because eating a little meat only makes you want more. And not only more meat, but also other high-fat foods—ice cream, butter, cakes, pies and so on," he says.

Dr. Ornish also cautions his patients to sharply curb their intake of alcohol, which suppresses the body's ability to burn fat, and refined sugar, which doesn't shut down your appetite the way complex carbohydrates do. "I've seen people gorge themselves on frozen nonfat yogurt, then wonder why their weight-loss efforts have stalled. They think that just because this frozen dessert has no fat it's okay. They forget it's loaded with sugar."

He does recommend that his patients take a multivitamin supplement every day as added insurance for maintaining good nutrition.

Why Cutting Fat Is Key

"If you reduce your fat intake to 10 percent, you really can eat more and weigh less." That's because you end up replacing fat calories with carbohydrate calories. And your body knows the difference.

Ounce for ounce, fat has more than twice the calories that protein or carbohydrates have. So you can eat the same amount of food but take in far fewer calories. What's more, says Dr. Ornish, your body readily converts fat calories into body fat; to convert carbohydrate or protein calories to body fat requires ten times the energy expenditure. Your body would rather burn these calories for energy than waste energy to store them.

Finally, complex carbohydrates, which have lots of fiber, fill you up fast. You feel full sooner, you stop eating sooner, and you take in fewer total calories.

Eat More Often, Not Less

146

One thing you may notice, however, is that after eating a high-carbohydrate meal, you feel hungry again sooner than after eating a high-fat meal. But that's okay, says Dr. Ornish. When you feel hungry, just eat. As long as you make smart food choices and eat only to the point of satiety, you're on the right track.

In fact, studies have shown that nibbling throughout the day has considerable weight-loss advantages, Dr. Ornish notes. When you maintain a somewhat steady intake of complex carbohydrates throughout the day, your blood sugar levels remain stable.

By contrast, when you eat sporadically and consume foods high in fat and sugar, your blood sugar soars and your body sends a surge of insulin to stabilize it. These insulin surges can work against a dieter's best intentions, says Dr. Ornish. Insulin steps up the body's release of an enzyme that promotes fat uptake from the bloodstream into body tissues. In other words, when insulin levels are high, you are more likely to build up body-fat stores.

For more information, read *Dr. Dean Ornish's Program for Reversing Heart Disease* and *Eat More, Weigh Less.*

Wipe Out Your Walking Woes   19

A walker's guide to shoes and foot maintenance.

You're feeling great. Over the last three months you've worked your way up to walking two miles a day. You wake up feeling more energetic. You've even started to drop some pounds.

The last thing you want is an injury that knocks you off your feet and puts a crimp in your exercise routine. True, walking is one of the safest and most effective ways to exercise. But many foot problems you've had all along may suddenly surface after you've started a regular walking program. So why not take steps now to protect yourself against potential problems before they break your stride?

On an average walking day, your feet carry 200 tons of weight. They're built to stand that pressure and more. But if you want them to keep carrying that load without pain or injury, you need to give them proper care and attention. And perhaps the most important step is to choose the right shoes.

Choose Your Shoes Carefully

"Shoes are made commercially. The foot is not made commercially," says Marc Lenet, D.P.M., chief of podiatry at University Hospital at the University of Maryland and Liberty Medical Center in Baltimore. Therein lies the challenge. Since you can't change your foot to fit a shoe, you have to choose a shoe that fits your foot. There are three specific things to look for in a shoe, says Lloyd Smith, D.P.M., past president of the American Academy of Podiatric Sports Medicine:

1. Cushioning ▶ "Every time you take a step, your foot hits the ground and a certain amount of impact is created," says Dr. Smith. So your goal is to find a shoe with plenty of cushioning to lessen that impact as much as possible. "You can feel confident that you've got adequate cushioning for fitness walking if you choose a shoe designed for walking, running, tennis or cross-training," he says.

Cushioning is so important that Long Beach, California, podiatrist John W. Pagliano, D.P.M., recommends adding a shock-absorbing insert to your walking shoes as you get older. "We all lose some of that fatty padding in the foot as we get older. This restores some of that cushioning." You can buy padded shoe inserts in most large drugstores.

148

2. Support ▶ Look for a shoe with a rigid heel that doesn't bend when you press on it, says Dr. Pagliano.

Then squeeze the top of the shoe in several places from toe to heel. If it's too soft, it won't hold your foot in place. But make sure the sole bends easily at the ball of the foot.

3. Fit ▶ All the cushioning and support in the world won't help if your shoes don't fit. So take these steps to guarantee a proper fit:

■ Try on shoes late in the day, when your feet are slightly swollen. "When you walk, your feet swell, so you want a shoe that is large enough to accommodate them during and after a long walk, not just in the shoe store," says Dr. Pagliano. "And wear the same type of socks you will wear with the shoes."

■ Follow Dr. Smith's rule of toe: "When the shoe is laced up, your heel shouldn't slip around inside the shoe and you should have enough room in the toes—say ¼ to ½ inch between the inside of the shoe and the tip of the longest toe."

■ Stand on tiptoe. To check the fit of the front of a new shoe, go up on tiptoe, recommends Annu Goel, D.P.M., a podiatrist in Alexandria, Virginia, and vice president of the American Association for Women Podiatrists. "When you go up on your toes, the front part of your foot, where it bends, should not be pinched. The shoe should feel comfortable and bend easily at the same point where the ball of your foot does. This puts weight on the front part of your foot and assures you that the shoe is not too narrow."

■ Look for snug heels—they're vital. "A good-fitting shoe cups your heel snugly, without pinching, offers support in the arch area and gives you room for your toes," says Dr. Goel. A snug heel is especially important for women, she says. "Women have proportionately narrower heels than men, so when they buy shoes that are wide enough in the front, their heels may come out of the shoe. If they try to fit the heel correctly, the front of the foot may be squeezed."

Instead of choosing between these two terrible options—a loose heel or crammed toes—decide which is

149
■

easier for you to correct. "There are two ways to do this," says Dr. Goel. "First, you can buy shoes that are wide enough up front and insert pads to make the heel snugger. I recommend having the store where the shoes are bought do it. Or a podiatrist can do it.

"The second strategy is to buy a shoe with a snug heel and have the front part of the shoe stretched. But generally this works only with shoes made of leather."

Don't settle for what the store has in stock if the fit isn't correct, says Dr. Goel. "A lot of stores don't carry all the widths, so I tell people to have the store order the correct width for them. Shoes should fit correctly in the store and not require breaking in."

And never ask for a specific size when you're in a shoe store. Instead, have both feet measured (while standing) anytime you shop for shoes.

Replace Your Shoes Every 500 Miles

"Lots of walkers come in with a problem," says Dr. Smith. "I ask about their shoes and they say, 'You know, I wear these shoes all the time; I've been wearing them for two years, and they're really comfortable.'

"I tell them, 'That's half your problem!' Walkers just don't seem to understand that if the shoes are worn out, they don't have the cushioning to protect their feet from the stresses of all the walking they're doing. All they can see is that the shoes don't have any holes in them and are still comfortable. But the midsole area is what disintegrates and weakens its support and cushioning—and you can't see that."

Since you can't actually see, or feel, how worn and weak your shoes have become, podiatrists recommend keeping track of how many miles you walk and replacing shoes regularly, regardless of how worn they appear. "The guideline we use for running," says Dr. Smith, "is 300 to 500 miles. For walking, you don't have quite as much stress generated, but many of the walking shoes are not as well cushioned as running shoes are, so I usually tell people to replace their shoes every 500 miles."

Is there a rule for breaking in walking shoes? "Most athletic shoes are almost broken in when you buy them. I wouldn't go out and walk an hour in a shoe I bought that day, however," says Dr. Smith. "I'd wear it around the house for a couple of hours a day for a few days."

Team Your Shoes with the Right Socks

While you're taking a careful look at your walking shoes, don't neglect your socks. "Perspiration is one of the biggest enemies of foot health when it sits there on the skin and is not removed properly," says Dr. Lenet. Warm sweat creates a breeding ground for infectious organisms. Then, while you're walking, the pores of the skin stretch and contract, making it easier for these organisms to penetrate the skin and cause trouble.

Dr. Lenet advises using socks that keep feet drier, as cotton-synthetic blends do, by wicking the moisture away from the surface of the skin. If you're going on a long hike, take along an extra pair of socks to change into.

Stretch Your Feet

Regular stretching is a vital part of walking for fitness, experts agree. It gets the blood flowing to all the muscles and tendons in your foot and makes your walking more injury free and comfortable. Start by walking for about five minutes to warm up. Then stretch the foot and lower-leg muscles. Stretch again after your walk.

The best stretch for walkers is the so-called wall push-up, says Dr. Smith. "Stand facing the wall, with one leg in front of the other. Keep the back foot flat and slowly bend the front leg as you hold your arms out against the wall for balance and support. You'll feel the pull in the back of your leg and in your Achilles tendon. Do this for about half a minute and then switch legs and repeat."

Give Your Feet a Treat

Those tired old dogs do a lot of work for us. If we give them some special attention, they'll return it tenfold in pleasure and hard work. Here are some recommendations:

■ Dr. Pagliano tells all his patients to wash their feet daily, smooth rough skin with a pumice stone and apply skin cream. "Use a stiff brush to clean the nail borders," he says. "I use an old toothbrush after every shower. This helps prevent fungus infections and ingrown nails—and it takes only a few seconds."

■ Regularly trimmed toenails are another essential for walkers, according to Dr. Pagliano. "Trim them with a clipper designed for toenails and leave a slightly rounded edge—but don't cut down the sides. If you trim to a sharp edge it could cut into the skin."

■ Don't overlook the value of massage. Dr. Goel says, "A foot massage at the end of the day is an excellent way to release tension."

Your Early Warning System

When it comes to walking injuries, everything starts small, says Dr. Lenet. But it doesn't always end small. One walker ignored a minor injury to her big toe. Instead of resting until the injury healed, she tried to "walk through the pain." She unconsciously compensated by shifting her weight off the injured toe and onto another part of her foot, which couldn't handle the added stress. A neuroma, or pinched nerve, developed over time and eventually required surgery.

To prevent small problems from escalating into large ones, it's essential to pay attention to your body's early warning signs. And the first sign of trouble is usually pain, which is not normal. You'd be amazed by the number of walkers who simply ignore this flashing light, says Dr. Smith. "Walkers, for some reason, often fail to make the connection between pain and their walking," he says.

But you can keep small injuries from turning into big ones if you recognize these early warning signs. "A lot of injuries are really subtle," says Dr. Smith. "You don't feel them until you're exercising. Or they sort of hurt a little bit during the day or the next day, and you're not really sure that the pain is coming from your walking or from something else. You have to pay attention to the pattern and make the connection."

You can expect a little transient discomfort from time to time, says Dr. Lenet: "a little muscle fatigue, a little pressure on a joint or nerve causing some temporary inflammation. There may be nothing to it. But if it persists, it could signal a problem."

Make Regular Inspections

"Regular self-examination of the feet is very important," says Dr. Lenet, because we can often see problems developing before we actually feel them as discomfort or pain. "At least by inspection we can observe any unusual changes, such as redness, swelling, heat, cracks in the skin or blisters."

"If you don't have any problems with frequent irritations with your toes or the bottoms of your feet, then you're doing okay," says Dr. Smith. "But if there's a spot on your foot that's always irritated, then there's probably an actual problem developing there. Shoes may be the culprit, or it may be the structure of your foot. In either case, you can do something."

What's your first step once you know you're having a problem? Is it in the direction of a podiatrist's office? Not necessarily. Depending on the problem, the first step may be to rest, or to apply some ice or a massage, or perhaps to go out and buy new shoes, or increase the cushioning of the old ones by inserting a cushion insole.

If you have diabetes or circulation problems, you should have every foot problem checked by your doctor or a podiatrist. Otherwise, you only need to visit a podiatrist if the pain is excruciating or persists for more than a couple of days—or if there are any large new bumps on your foot.

The American Podiatric Medical Association (APMA) is an organization of nearly 10,000 doctors of podiatric medicine dedicated to improving the quality of foot care. For a free brochure on a variety of foot-care concerns, call the APMA at (800) FOOTCARE.

20   Knock Out Knee Pain

Easy exercises for easing aches, restoring strength and improving flexibility.

If you think memory is the first casualty of aging, you're wrong. It's the knee. In fact, the knee can lose up to half its strength in just two decades.

That's no surprise. The human knee—that poor, run-down joint—has more burdens to bear than a counselor at a camp for rambunctious kids. It has the largest weight-bearing surface of any joint in the body and, when functioning at normal capacity, is subjected to stresses far in excess of any other joint. No wonder so many knees end up in therapy.

Not that therapy always works. The knee's a repeat offender—hurt once, it has an even greater chance of getting hurt again.

An estimated 50 million Americans suffer from some sort of knee pain or injury. A problem in the joint may not just limit itself to that one spot, either. By decreasing a person's activity level, knee trouble may lead to weight gain and decreased cardiovascular health, which can potentially snowball into an increased risk for developing heart disease.

There's a strategy, however, that may keep knees pain free and throw a roadblock in front of the snowball. Resistance training may very well be the ultimate knee saver by offering preventive protection for both healthy and troubled knees. We're talking "rehab" and "prehab."

Protective Rehab

Usually knee experts recommend resistance training after knee trouble begins. After serious injury or surgery, a period of rest and range-of-motion therapy follows. Then comes the muscle strengthening.

The hamstring muscles and the quadriceps muscles (on the back and front of the thigh) are the key to successful rehabilitation and healthier knees. They provide strong support for the knee—the quadriceps with its four "heads" that attach over the joint and the hamstring muscles that attach along the sides of the knee. (Note: The hamstrings are tendons that attach the hamstring muscles to the sides of the knee.)

It's vital for knee health that the quadriceps and hamstring muscles aren't just strong but balanced as well (we'll get to that later). Whether it's a torn ligament or osteoarthritis, training these muscles plays a vital role in returning you to normal function.

Loathsome Ligaments ▶ Ligaments play a huge role in protecting and stabilizing the knee. Within the knee joint, two strong ligaments crisscross each other to hold the joint together. These ligaments are most vulnerable to injury in sudden-stop sports like soccer or football. But many times, the troubled tissue may just wear with age. Depending on the severity of the problem, options range from rest to surgical ligament replacement.

"Most people never know they have any problems with the ligament until it pops," says Thomas D. Rizzo Jr., M.D., co-director of the Sports Medicine Center at the Mayo Clinic in Rochester, Minnesota. "Over many years, you may experience repeated, mild injuries to the ligament, until finally the coup de grace comes when you overdo it."

Once that pop occurs, strength training becomes an effective therapy for dealing with the aftermath, usually as part of a more comprehensive rehabilitative program. Simple exercises (which you'll learn later) that strengthen the quadriceps and hamstring muscles are helpful in building a stable fortress around the trouble tissue—protecting it not only from further injury but also from surgery.

One study, for instance, looked at 26 patients with ruptured front knee ligaments, all eligible for surgery. After undertaking a three- to six-month period of muscle training, 22 of the group were satisfied enough with their improvement in function and activity level that they were able to bypass surgery. Many experienced less swelling, pain and "giving way" following the exercise period.

In another study following 61 patients with old ligament injuries, all were considered for surgery but instead underwent a three-month strength-training program. Although 40 percent of the patients eventually underwent ligament reconstruction, the remaining 60 percent had almost normal knee function even five years after they finished the muscle-building program. And in later research from the same doctors, 53 patients troubled by old tears and candidates for surgery took part in a similar strengthening program. Improvement in strength and performance was so great that the majority of the group declined surgery.

If strength training isn't tapped to preserve muscle after ligament injury, things can only get worse. Inactivity opens the door to muscle atrophy. But this atrophy no longer becomes just a consequence. It actually becomes a cause of more damage by directly increasing knee instability and malalignment. This may not only lead to or accelerate osteoarthritis but may also cause ligament and cartilage damage, discomfort and disuse of the knee. And this increases muscle atrophy even more.

Researchers stress that this diabolical domino effect can be stopped without going under the surgeon's knife. Simply by strengthening the muscles to prevent wasting, the cycle sputters and recovery begins.

156

Cranky Kneecaps ▶ The patella, or kneecap, is the protective bone at the front of the knee and one of three bones that comprise the knee joint. It's the hot spot for the most common kind of knee pain, called chondromalacia. Doctors often group this kind of kneecap pain and others under one umbrella called patellofemoral-pain syndrome. Most pain results from uneven or excess pressure on the kneecap during activity or overuse due to heavy leg impact—from thumping aerobics or running.

In one study, isometric (fixed exercises that don't involve any movement of the joint or limb) and other strength-training techniques were used to combat kneecap pain. Women worked out three times a week for four weeks, using Velcro sandbags to strengthen their thighs and stretch their hamstring muscles. Although pain measurements remained unchanged, their quadriceps strength and hamstring-muscle strength improved significantly, allowing them to take part in more activities with improved function. The bolstered muscles let them compensate for their troubled kneecaps.

And for other kinds of kneecap pain, simple isometrics have been used in cases where the people can't deal with full-on lifting. Patients simply flex their quadriceps for short spans of time, placing their own hand on the muscle. That way they can feel the muscle tightening, making them aware exactly what the exercise is doing and where it's doing it.

Painful Osteoarthritis ▶ Research suggests that osteoarthritis can occur in roughly 44 to 70 percent of people over 55. Ten percent of people in that group find their daily functions limited by it.

Studies have shown that aerobic exercise boosts cardiovascular health in people suffering from this kind of wear-and-tear knee problem, but rarely is any improvement seen in muscular strength. "And although aerobic endurance is important, we've found that muscle, not the cardiovascular system, is really the limiting factor as we grow older," says Nadine M. Fisher, Ed.D., assistant professor of rehabilitation medicine at the University of Buffalo in New York. That's why Dr. Fisher turns to strength training in her rehabilitation regimen, with dramatic results.

157

In her latest study, involving 80 people with knee osteoarthritis, 90 percent experienced less pain, 85 percent had improved muscle strength and endurance, and 95 percent had increased functional capacity after a three-month exercise and therapy program. The exercises started out with isometrics and gradually worked up to full resistance-training exercises that again targeted the quadriceps and hamstring muscles.

"Once you build up the muscles around the knee joint, they can absorb the shock from walking and other activities, so you can do more without having pain in your knee," says Dr. Fisher. More important for older folks, the exercises may make a big impact by preventing big impacts. "These exercises help to train the person's neurological system to react faster," she says. "This helps prevent falls and maintain balance, which reduces chances for broken bones."

Dr. Fisher doesn't know if the exercises are actually changing the nature of the disease, but by building the muscles, people have been able to create an active detour around the obstacle of illness. "Our patients walk straighter, are more flexible and realize they're not as limited as they once thought they were," she says. One of the study participants had given up fishing because his knee joints prevented him from lugging his boat up a steep hill.

"Rather than selling his boat, he's back out fishing," says Dr. Fisher.

Protective "Prehab"

So strength training can treat knee disorders. But what about prevention? Research pitting muscle training against future incidence of knee problems is scarce, though most researchers think the same strengthening exercises geared for making bad knees better may also keep good knees from going bad.

"If we can rehabilitate an injury using these exercises, it's our rationale that we can prevent these injuries with those same exercises," says Lyle L. Micheli, M.D., past president of the American College of Sports

Medicine and associate professor of orthopedics at Harvard University.

Bank on a Balance ▶ Muscles come in pairs. Each one is balanced by another that performs an opposite function. For example, the quadriceps support the movement of the leg while you extend it, and the hamstring muscles support it while you bend it. To prevent knee problems, be an equal-opportunity muscle flexer.

"Joints were designed through evolution to have a balance of muscle around them," says M. Solomonow, Ph.D., professor of orthopedic surgery and director of the bioengineering section at the Louisiana State Medical Center in New Orleans. "If either of these two muscles becomes too strong, it can cause an inordinate pull on one side of the knee joint, making it vulnerable to extra stress and injury."

The lopsided leg is no rarity. "Generally, most people's quadriceps are about 50 percent stronger than their hamstrings," says Dr. Rizzo.

In order to keep one muscle from overpowering another and causing abnormal shear-type stresses on the joint, researchers advocate strengthening the hamstring muscles so as to become equal to the quadriceps. "Strengthening the leg muscles without restoring a balance between them is simply asking for trouble," says Dr. Solomonow.

You can specifically train each muscle—with leg extensions for the thighs and hamstring curls on a weight machine. Dr. Rizzo, however, thinks it's best to exercise them all at once. "We found that strengthening the muscles together may actually be better on the knee," he says.

The key is to use exercises that move all the parts of the leg in concert: the hip, knee and ankle. "The hamstring muscles and quadriceps would work together in a functional and appropriate manner without stressing the knee," says Dr. Rizzo. "You don't have one muscle from one side putting abnormal shear-type stresses on the joint."

Squats or lunges are examples of these types of exercises. But there are simpler, less strenuous exercises that do the trick, too. "Stationary cycling and stair climbing are both effective exercises that strengthen the knees without causing too much shear on the knee," says Dr. Micheli.

Start Sooner, Not Later ▶ You may be feeling just the first twinges of arthritis in your knees, but don't put off a protective exercise program. In fact, experts say, the earlier the better.

"Although there is no definitive evidence yet, the right kind of strengthening exercises may prolong the time before arthritis becomes a problem," says Dr. Fisher. "By building the muscles around the knee for support, use of medications, knee replacements and other serious procedures may be greatly reduced. And you may be able to live pain-free for a lot longer."

Hand the Ligament a Lifesaver ▶ You don't have to be a pro ballplayer to be vulnerable to a ligament injury. Ligaments answer to time. In fact, this tissue can weaken tremendously with age, severely depleting the load-carrying capacity of an average knee by the time you reach 40.

Strength training, though, may play a role in preventing this decline. "An exercise program using light weights with a high number of repetitions, when done carefully, may help prevent this age-related weakening from occurring," says Freddie H. Fu, M.D., professor of orthopedic surgery and chief of the Sportsmedicine Division at the University of Pittsburgh Medical Center, who is researching age-related ligament damage. "By building up the muscles around the joint, you may offer a wall of protection around the ligament."

Knee-Power Strategies

It would be nice to have one set of exercises to fit all knees. But we don't. Each knee is different, and since you have only two, you don't want to put them under unnecessary strain.

The exercise menu presented here, however, offers

excellent options for stretching and building the quadriceps and hamstring muscles. Because the calf muscle also adds some support to the knee, we've thrown in an exercise for that, too.

For a healthy person, these exercises offer potent protection; for a person with a bum knee, the milder exercises make great therapy. If you're already saddled with knee problems, see a sportsmedicine therapist or orthopedist first to decide how much you can do and how often. People with serious ligament damage should shy away from anything that puts heavy stress on the area.

And even if you have mild ligament problems, be extra careful. Exercises that target the quadriceps tend to put tremendous pressure on the ligaments. If they're already injured, the exercises can make matters worse. "The problem is, if you skip the exercises, the muscle atrophies, and then you've got another problem," says Dr. Solomonow. His advice to those with ligament problems is to do the exercises but shorten the range of motion considerably. It may also be worthwhile to skip resistance exercises that move the joint and start out with simple isometrics.

And listen to your body. "The normal discomfort— stiffness, an aching feeling— should go away as you get farther into the workout," says Dr. Rizzo. "But if the pain gets worse as you progress or causes you to limp or protect a joint, then lay off."

Hamstring-Muscle Stretch ▶ Extend your right leg straight out with the toes pointed up. Bend your left leg in and touch the sole of your foot to the inside of your right thigh. Lean forward from the hips. The back of your thigh should feel tight but not painful. Hold for 30 seconds to three minutes and then switch legs. Stretch each leg once.

Quadriceps Stretch ▶ Lie on your side and grasp the ankle of the top leg with your hand. Pull your foot toward your buttocks. Keep your hips forward, so you stretch the front of the thigh and not the ankle. You can also do this stretch while standing.

Leg and Thigh Extensions ▶ Get a rope and stand on it with your knees flexed 90 degrees. Grasp the rope firmly with your hands at your sides and your arms hanging straight down. Keeping your body erect, try to straighten your legs by lifting upward.

Leg Press ▶ Sit in a doorway with your back against one side of the door frame and your feet against the bottom of the other side. Grasp the door frame behind your head and try to extend your legs by pushing your feet against the frame.

Leg Curl ▶ At your dresser, pull out the lower drawer slightly. Lying on your stomach, with your knees slightly bent, hook your heels under the bottom of the drawer. Try to pull your heels up toward your head, pulling against the tension of the drawer.

Wall Sit ▶ This targets the quadriceps. Stand three feet from a wall and lean back against it. Squat until your thighs are perpendicular to the wall, as though you're sitting on an invisible chair. Hold this position for 30 seconds. Build up to a set of five two-minute wall sits.

Front Lunge ▶ Stand with your head up, your back straight and your feet 14 inches apart. Step forward as far as possible with your right leg until your upper right thigh is almost parallel to the floor. Keep your lower leg straight. Then step back to the starting position. Repeat with the left leg. This can be done with weights—just hold them straight down at your sides.

To get the inner thigh, try a side lunge. Stand erect with your hands on your hips. Keep your back straight with your head up and your feet close together. Step to the side with your left leg as far as possible, with your knee bent, until your upper thigh is almost parallel to floor. Keep your right leg straight. Then step back to the starting position. Repeat with the other leg.

Quadriceps Extensions ▶ Sit on a leg-extension machine with your feet under the footpad. Raise the weight until your legs are two-thirds of the way up. Let the foot pad back down and repeat ten times for three sets. Here's how to do this at home: Sit in a chair with your legs bent at the knees. With ankle weights (up to ten pounds), raise your leg and hold for six seconds, then rest. Switch legs. Repeat ten times for three sets. Don't extend your legs fully if you have ligament injuries, because it may cause more problems. Instead, you can do the last 30 degrees (about six to eight inches) of the exercises.

Hamstring-Muscle Builders ▶ On a thigh-and-knee machine, lie on your stomach and hook your heels under the hamstring attachment. Then slowly bend your knees, bringing your feet toward your buttocks. Pause briefly, then lower the weight slowly. To do this at home, stand braced against a wall, bend your knee and lift your leg off the ground behind you (you can wear ankle weights). Hold for a count of ten. Perform three sets of ten repetitions with each leg.

Standing Dumbbell Toe Raise ▶ This exercise helps build the calf muscles. Hold the weight in your left hand, letting it hang down at your side, with your palm in. Then step up with the ball of your right foot on a platform raised a few inches off the ground and about two feet away from the wall. Place your right hand against the wall. Make sure your back is straight, with your head up and your right knee locked. Hook your right foot behind your left heel. Don't let your hips move backward or forward. Then raise up on your toes as high as you can. Hold that position for a moment, then return again to your starting position. Switch legs and weight, then repeat.

21   Cholesterol Breakthroughs

Raising this number can lower your risk for heart diease.

Good news! The results of your latest screening test say your total cholesterol's down to a heart-healthy sub-200. But before you let loose a sigh of relief, find out how much heart-protecting HDL cholesterol you have in your blood. The reason is that a growing pile of evidence—and a crowd of the world's experts—say total cholesterol readings don't tell the whole story. According to them, your total cholesterol combined with your HDL level is an even better indicator of your heart health.

Since 1988, when the first cholesterol-screening guidelines were issued, you were considered home free if you kept your total cholesterol under 200. Only if you topped that were your lipid (blood fat) levels scrutinized further. And even then the emphasis was on lowering the level of artery-clogging LDL cholesterol. HDL was virtually ignored.

But at least four studies involving thousands of people—including the landmark Framingham Heart Study—have found that the lower your HDL level, the higher your risk for heart disease. In fact, in most of those studies, HDL levels were better at predicting future heart attacks than total cholesterol alone and LDL cholesterol.

To be sure, your risk of heart attack drops along with your total cholesterol. "If your cholesterol is under 150, you have nothing to worry about," says William Castelli, M.D., director of the Framingham Heart Study, a study of a Massachusetts community to determine risk factors for heart disease. "But we know that many people with total cholesterol levels between 150 and 200 have heart attacks. The only way to find the people most likely to have heart attacks is to measure HDL. HDL measurements are almost three times better than LDL

164

measurements at predicting heart disease when the cholesterol is between 200 and 240—the range in which most heart attacks occur in our country."

Indeed, in one study, doctors checked the arteries of 1,084 people with cholesterol levels of less than 200 to look for evidence of heart disease. Angiograms—x-rays showing the inside of the arteries—revealed that 690 of them had telltale narrowing of at least one major heart vessel. Judging by their total cholesterol readings alone, doctors had no reason to suspect heart disease. But here's a revealing statistic: Sixty percent of the group of 690—414 people—had HDL levels of less than 35.

Another study looked at the lipids of 212 people who had heart attacks, bypass surgery and/or angioplasty (a procedure used to unblock clogged arteries). Nearly half of them had total cholesterol of less than 200. But 52 percent of that group had HDL levels below 35—and many were under 30.

"That means that if we just look at total cholesterol, we're missing people whose total cholesterol is rather low but who also have low HDL levels—a pattern that's seen in up to 20 percent of heart attack patients," says Basil Rifkind, M.D., chief of the Lipid Metabolism and Atherosclerosis Branch of the National Heart, Lung and Blood Institute.

The Magic Ratio

The millions of potential heart attack victims going untreated has led experts to rethink their emphasis on total cholesterol readings as the sole screen for heart disease. In fact, the National Cholesterol Education Project—a government group that sets cholesterol-screening guidelines—will most likely include a new recommendation that your HDL be measured every time you're screened for total cholesterol.

The new guidelines are expected to recommend shooting for an HDL level over 40. That's the minimum, according to the experts. "I think 50 or above should be the goal—especially for women, because research suggests that HDL is slightly more protective in women than in men, although we don't really understand why," says Trudy Bush, Ph.D., associate professor of epidemiology at Johns Hopkins School of Hygiene and Public Health in Baltimore.

HDL is shorthand for high-density lipoproteins—tiny globules of fat created in the liver. They're suspected of being your body's bouncers—rousting LDL cholesterol from your arteries, where it tends to loiter, causing dangerous blockages. That process, dubbed "reverse cholesterol transport," is what many researchers attribute HDL's heart-protecting capabilities to.

To help figure out where your HDL level should be to minimize your risk of heart disease, look at your total cholesterol. "If it's over 150, the simplest way—and the best way—to determine your risk is to divide your total cholesterol by your HDL measurement," Dr. Castelli says. That gives you a magic number—the ratio of total cholesterol to HDL cholesterol, which actually proved to be the best predictor of heart attack in the Framingham and the Physicians' Health studies.

Say your reading is 160, but your HDL level's holding steady at 30—that gives you a rounded-off ratio of 5.3 to 1, or just 5.3. Now research suggests that anything at 4.5 or higher means you could be at risk. If you are, your doctor should look at the levels of other blood fats—particularly LDL cholesterol and triglycerides—to get a better picture of your risk profile. Then you can work on strategies to change it.

On the flip side, HDL measurements can also help identify the fraction of people who have danger-zone total cholesterol levels but who aren't at increased risk of heart attack. Alarms automatically sound when you get a total cholesterol reading of 300. But if your HDL's 75, you've got a 4:1 ratio, well within heart-healthy boundaries. Looking at total cholesterol alone, though, you'd be in for a lifetime of cholesterol-lowering drug therapy.

Shaping Up Your Profile

166
∎

The impact of lowering the levels of LDL cholesterol on heart disease risk have been well established with comprehensive scientific studies. Similar studies on dropping heart disease risk by upping HDL are just now yielding results. In fact, a recent analysis of the major cholesterol-and-heart-disease studies suggests that for every point you raise your HDL, your risk of heart disease drops 2 to 3 percent.

Manipulating your total-cholesterol-to-HDL ratio— through either raising HDL or lowering total cholesterol—might bring you even bigger benefits. An analysis of the data from the Physicians' Health Study suggested that a drop of one unit in the total-cholesterol-to-HDL ratio may cut your risk of heart attack by 53 percent. That means that if your total cholesterol level is 200 and your HDL is 40, you have a ratio of 5. Raising your HDL level to 50 would bring your ratio down a full point—to a heart-safe 4—with just half the risk.

There are a number of ways to boost your HDL levels. The most dramatic increases are seen in people in drug therapy. But HDL-raising drugs are reserved for people who also have other heart disease risk factors, like elevated LDLs, high triglycerides or already established heart disease. And they're prescribed to those people only after they fail to respond to lifestyle changes.

A drink or two of alcohol a day has also been linked to higher HDL levels. But when researchers try to establish a direct cause-and-effect relationship by giving humans alcohol and measuring HDL in the aftermath, they're unable to produce a consistent result. Alcohol, because it's processed by your body like fat, can also add excess pounds. And being overweight is strongly associated with low HDL.

Here are the best ways to boost your HDL levels, according to the latest research.

Take a Stroll

A number of studies have suggested that heartbeat-accelerating aerobic exercise, like speedwalking, running and cycling, can jack up HDL levels as much as 10 to 20 percent. But the most recent news from research laboratories is that you may not have to sweat bullets to see your

HDL levels rise. *Prevention* reported on a study of 59 women divided into four groups. They all walked three miles a day three to four times a week, but at different paces. One group walked at 12 minutes per mile (fast), another walked at 15 minutes per mile (brisk) and the third strolled at 20 minutes per mile. The fourth group remained sedentary. While the women who walked faster were in better cardiovascular shape than the strollers, each group saw the same 6 percent rise in HDL. That meant their heart disease risk fell 18 percent.

"The bottom line is that people who just exercise regularly, not necessarily very hard, might be able to expect some rise in HDL cholesterol," says Kerry Stewart, Ed.D., assistant professor of medicine and clinical exercise physiologist at Johns Hopkins University

DEADLY COMBINATIONS

Your HDL cholesterol level could be the key to what's shaking out to be a deadly combination—low HDL levels and high triglycerides.

Triglycerides are a conglomeration of four different fats transported in the body by protein envelopes called very-low-density lipoproteins (VLDL). VLDLs come in two varieties—a large, benign kind that can't lodge in artery walls and a small, dense, heart disease–causing version. Elevated triglyceride levels don't necessarily mean you're at increased risk—if, that is, you have the large, buoyant kind. But there's no way to tell which type of VLDL you have unless you look at your HDL cholesterol measurement.

"If your HDL is 40 or lower and your triglycerides get over 100, you're starting to put out the small, dense VLDL," says William Castelli, M.D., director of the Framingham Heart Study. "If your triglycerides hit 150, you're really into the dangerous territory of the small, dense, artery-clogging particles."

In a five-year study of 4,081 men aged 40 to 55, the group with HDL levels of less than 42 and triglyceride

in Baltimore. "But most of the evidence suggests that the more exercise you do and the harder you do it, the more likely you are to see a rise in HDL."

Although they don't know for sure, researchers suspect that the action of an enzyme called lipoprotein lipase is accelerated when you exercise. That causes a faster turnover of fat, resulting in less lipid buildup in the blood.

Get Rid of Your Girth

If you're overweight, losing those extra pounds is probably your best way to boost your HDL levels. "People who are more than 30 percent over their ideal body weight generally have very low HDL levels," says Dr. Bush. Indeed, in a study of 491 middle-aged women,

levels greater than 200 had almost twice as many heart attacks as the group whose HDL levels were equal to or greater than 42. Ten percent of the men in that same study also had the "lipid triad"—low HDL, high triglycerides and high LDL levels. They were four times as likely to have a heart attack as the men who had an inherited disorder characterized by elevated LDL levels—who are already at high risk of heart attack.

Even riskier, though, is the combination of a big belly, high triglycerides, low HDL, high blood sugar and high blood pressure—"the American disease par excellence," Dr. Castelli calls it. "In the Framingham Study, that syndrome produced twice as many heart attacks as any other lipid syndrome, and it's very common—about one-fourth of the population has it," he says. "It's characterized by triglycerides over 150, HDL levels under 40, obesity around the midsection, blood sugar over 100 and borderline or high blood pressure. And it's totally preventable through lifestyle changes—particularly diet and exercise."

169

the group with the highest body-mass index (an indicator of excess weight, calculated by dividing body weight by height) had, on average, HDL levels 15 points lower than the women with the lowest body-mass index.

Most research suggests that you'll see the sharpest surge in HDL with a combination of diet and exercise. In one study, 231 moderately overweight men and women were divided into three groups. One group didn't change its eating and exercise regimen, and one went on a low-fat, high-carbohydrate diet. The third ate the same slim-down diet but walked briskly or jogged 25 to 45 minutes a day three days a week. After a year on the program, the HDL levels of the exercise-plus-diet group were 11 percent higher than those of the dieters alone.

Overall, women didn't fare as well as men in this study. On the weight-loss diet alone, their HDLs actually fell, which is not unusual. "It's just as important for women to exercise as it is for men," says Dr. Bush. "Exercise helps to counteract the HDL drop caused by a low-fat diet alone."

Exercise can help increase lean body mass and decrease fat mass, Dr. Stewart says. "And the improvement in the ratio of lean to fat, especially if the fat comes out of the upper body, seems to result in higher HDL levels."

And research suggests that you not only have to lose fat, you also have to lose it in the right place to boost your HDL levels. A number of studies have linked low HDL levels—and higher heart disease risk—with excess upper-body weight. In a preliminary study of 13 obese premenopausal women, the women who lost the most total body fat—especially in the abdominal area—after a 14-month aerobic exercise plan showed the biggest HDL increases and LDL decreases. When researchers measured the activity of the fat-burning enzyme, lipoprotein lipase, they found it accelerated the most in those women who lost the most weight.

How do you get rid of a belt-busting belly? Spot-reduction isn't the answer. "People think that if they do sit-ups, they'll lose fat in their bellies. That's not true—they'll just develop hard muscles under the fat," Dr. Stewart says. "In order to lose the fat, you have to diet and exercise. Then the fat will come off in the spots where it has accumulated the most."

How much weight should you lose? "Weight goals are a tough issue, because your ideal body weight depends on the size of your frame," Dr. Bush says. "Talk to your doctor, a nutritionist or a dietitian to help you determine your weight-loss goals."

Stay Away from Smoke

It's well established that cigarette smokers have lower HDL levels, although it's not yet understood why. And now there's preliminary evidence that you may not have to be a smoker yourself to suffer the HDL-lowering effect of cigarettes. A study of 391 students in suburban New York showed that nonsmoking students who were exposed to high levels of secondhand smoke had almost 7 percent lower HDL cholesterol levels than nonsmoking students who had less exposure to smoke.

"Passive smoke definitely has an effect on people— the biggest impact, of course, is on lung cancer," Dr. Castelli says. "But smoking definitely pushes down HDL levels, so passive smoking may do the same thing."

Consider Estrogen Therapy

Between ages 45 and 55, women's HDL levels plateau, while their LDL and total cholesterol levels go up. Experts believe that some of these changes are due to less estrogen—the female hormone—circulating through the body during and after menopause. "No one knows how estrogen therapy keeps HDL levels high," Dr. Bush says. "but when you put a woman on a typical dose of oral estrogen, LDL is lowered about 10 to 12 percent and HDL increases by about 16 to 20 percent." That could translate into a substantial dip in your heart disease risk.

Women in the Framingham Study whose HDL levels increased by 10 percent saw a 40 to 50 percent reduction in risk. The evidence has led experts to recommend estrogen therapy as a first-line treatment for women with low HDL or high LDL levels. "But any woman

171
■

who's considering estrogen replacement therapy has to answer a whole list of questions with her physician," says Marianne Legato, M.D., associate professor of clinical medicine at Columbia University College of Physicians and Surgeons in New York City and author of *The Female Heart.* "Only after those questions are answered is it appropriate to even think about taking estrogen."

Some studies have linked estrogen therapy to breast cancer—other studies have not. So if you have a personal or family history of breast cancer, discuss your options with your doctor. It's much more well established that estrogen increases your risk of uterine cancer. Adding progestin (another female hormone) cancels estrogen's

A HEALTHY DROP IN HDL?

When it comes to HDL, the higher, the better—right? Not always. People who eat ultra-low-fat, high-carbohydrate diets, and vegetarians, run consistently low on HDL, but few of them develop heart disease. In fact, the tried-and-true heart-healthy diet often results in a slight decrease in HDL levels. In one study, 19 women ate a typical American diet of 37 percent of calories from fat—most of it saturated—44 percent from carbohydrates and 19 percent from protein. After one month, they were switched to a strict diet designed to reduce total cholesterol—21 percent of calories from fat, 59 percent from carbohydrates and 19 percent from protein. Two months of that feeding regimen resulted in a 12 percent drop in HDL, which leveled off to 5 percent after five months on the diet.

No one is quite sure what causes HDL to slide downward in response to the state-of-the-heart healthy diet. "But if eating a very-low-fat, high-carbohydrate diet makes your HDL levels drop, your LDL and total cholesterol levels usually go down faster—and your total-cholesterol-to-HDL ratio improves," says William

capability to cause uterine cancer, but it may not result in the same HDL-boosting benefits. "Instead of increasing HDL by about 16 to 20 percent, you may increase it 10 to 12 percent with estrogen and progestin combined," Dr. Bush says. "But if a woman hasn't had her uterus removed with a hysterectomy, she needs progestin to protect the uterine lining from cancer."

Hormone replacement therapy also increases levels of triglycerides in your body, but according to Dr. Castelli, they're the "good" triglycerides, not the type that cause heart disease. So higher triglycerides as a result of estrogen therapy aren't likely to affect your heart disease risk.

Castelli, M.D., director of the Framingham Heart Study. Indeed, the women saw a decrease in total cholesterol of 7 percent and an 11 percent drop in LDL over the five months of the study.

People who forgo meat and go for grains, vegetables and fruits instead also see their HDL drop—without a corresponding rise in heart disease risk. "There are many different reasons why people have low HDL," says Basil Rifkind, M.D., of the National Heart, Lung and Blood Institute. "Some people have them because they eat healthy diets. Then there are people whose low HDL levels are connected to cigarette smoking, being overweight or not exercising. We need more research to help us understand why low HDL is a risk factor for some people but not for others."

So despite a potential drop in HDL with a diet that's low in fat and high in complex carbohydrates, experts still say that's the way to eat if you want to lose weight and gain a healthy heart. And there's little reason to be concerned if your vegetarian diet leads to lower HDL.

Hormone therapy has some other side effects that are less dangerous but still unpleasant. You may experience breast tenderness, nausea or weight gain while you're taking estrogen. And the estrogen/progestin combination may cause menstrual-period–like bleeding. For now, experts suggest that the best decision for or against estrogen therapy is on a case-by-case basis, with your physician's input.

Try Niacin

This B vitamin is well known as a total cholesterol slasher and an HDL stimulant. It's so cardiac- and cost-effective, in fact, that it's often doctors' first choice when they're treating people whose cholesterol levels haven't responded to diet, exercise, smoking cessation and other lifestyle changes. In a study of 34 men with heart disease and very low levels of HDL (many below 30), three months of niacin therapy resulted in a 30 percent increase in HDL levels. Previous, larger-scale trials have produced similar results. Niacin short-circuits LDL production in your liver. That means less of the artery-clogging stuff is floating free in your arteries, where it's likely to accumulate.

The average dose of niacin it took to get such a gain in HDL levels was 2,400 milligrams—substantially higher than the U.S. Recommended Daily Allowance of 20 milligrams. Niacin at that dosage is considered to be a drug—not a vitamin. Doctors reserve its use, along with other cholesterol-lowering drugs, for people with markedly low HDL levels in combination with other heart disease risk factors. Such large amounts of niacin should not be taken without your doctor's supervision. People with stomach ulcers, liver dysfunction, diabetes or gouty arthritis are not good candidates for niacin therapy because it aggravates those conditions. It may also have other side effects, such as stomach cramps, skin flushing, itching and tingling. But timed-release niacin, housed in a wax casing, seems to have eliminated those problems.

Consider Vitamin C

Several studies from researchers at the USDA Human Nutrition Research Center on Aging at Tufts University in Boston indicate that the higher the level of vitamin C in your blood, the higher your HDL level. Blood vitamin C levels and HDL levels were tested in 1,372 men and women. Those who had the highest levels of vitamin C in their blood had 10 percent higher HDL levels than those with the lowest vitamin C levels.

"There may be an effect of vitamin C on HDL levels, but it's far from conclusive," says Paul Jacques, Sc.D., epidemiologist at the research center and author of the study. "Based on our research, people who consume 180 milligrams or above of vitamin C each day have 5 to 10 percent higher HDL levels than people with low amounts of vitamin C in their diets. That's not a dramatic difference, but it could translate to a substantial reduction in heart attack risk in a large population."

There have been few studies, though, in which people were fed vitamin C to observe the direct effect of the nutrient on their HDL levels. The studies done to date have been either too small or too flawed to yield any concrete conclusions, Dr. Jacques says. In the meantime, consuming 180 milligrams of vitamin C a day—three times the Recommended Dietary Allowance of 60—won't do you any harm.

Try a Different Oral Contraceptive

Birth control pills—like the hormone pills taken by many postmenopausal women—are combinations of estrogen and progestin, but oral contraceptives contain much more progestin, which has an effect on lipids opposite to that of estrogen: It lowers HDL and raises LDL.

"Before you begin taking the Pill, you should have a complete cholesterol profile check," Dr. Legato says. "If your total cholesterol is over 220 or your triglycerides are over 190 (after three measurements), then you should find an alternative birth control method until they're brought into normal range."

Once you've started on the Pill, have your cholesterol and triglyceride levels checked after the first three months, and again after the first year to make sure the levels are under control. "If you're having problems with your lipids while you're on oral contraceptives, talk to your doctor about trying another pill with a different progestin," Dr. Bush says. "Norethindrone and medroxyprogesterone acetate—other progestins—may have less effect on your cholesterol and triglycerides than norgestrel, another type of progestin."

Switch Beta-Blockers

Beta-blockers are drugs commonly prescribed to treat high blood pressure, chest pain, irregular heartbeats and migraine. They block the sites on your body tissues where neurotransmitters—chemicals released from nerve endings—attach, increasing your heartbeat and dilating blood vessels. That's how they slow your heartbeat, hold down your blood pressure and help prevent migraine headaches.

Researchers don't quite know why, but a type of beta-blocker known as a nonselective beta-blocker may lower your HDL level and increase your triglycerides. Talk to your doctor about switching to a cardioselective beta-blocker. Cardioselective beta-blockers work only on the heart and don't seem to lower HDL cholesterol.

Make Your Fat Mono

We know from reams of scientific research that reducing the amount of fat in your diet can significantly reduce your risk of heart disease and help you drop the pounds you need to see an HDL gain. Many experts agree that, to protect yourself, you need to reduce your fat intake to 25 percent of your calories.

And opting for monounsaturated fats (prevalent in foods like olive oil) may actually increase your HDL levels, according to research. Researchers put 46 men and 32 women on a diet that drew about 36 percent of calories from sunflower oil—a polyunsaturated fat—for

12 weeks. Then they switched their source of fat to olive oil. After 16 weeks on the olive-oil diet, the men saw a 17 percent increase in HDL. And the women saw their HDL levels shoot up 30 percent after 28 weeks. Their total-cholesterol-to-HDL ratios fell, too. The men's dropped 12 percent and the women's dropped 17 percent after they switched to olive oil.

"That suggests that diets high in monounsaturated fats may protect you from heart disease," Dr. Bush says. "So if you're going to eat fat, it's a good idea to substitute monos for other fats."

Get Hooked on Fish

Studies measuring the effects of the omega-3 fatty acids in fish like tuna, mackerel, salmon and sardines on HDL have yielded mixed results.

A recent review of the research says the average increase in HDL is 3 percent and some studies suggest that you could see as much as a 12 percent increase, but the fishy fats also cause dramatic dips in triglycerides. Eating the equivalent of seven ounces of fish a day cut triglycerides by more than 50 percent in one study. That's quite a mound of mackerel—but you don't need to eat that much if you decrease other sources of fat in your diet, because you'll be attacking HDL and triglycerides on two fronts.

"One of the 'magic bullets' against heart disease could be fish," Dr. Castelli says. "The societies whose diets emphasize fish have the lowest heart attack rate."

Fish-oil supplements may help you get your omega-3's, but don't take fish-oil capsules unless you're under your doctor's supervision. They may contain high amounts of vitamins A and D. And they cause abnormalities in blood sugar control, so people with diabetes should avoid using them.

Learn to Relax

A number of studies suggest that people who have high-stress lifestyles or who have a driven, hostile, type-

A personality have poor lipid profiles and higher risk of heart disease and heart attack. In fact, stress reduction is an essential part of a revolutionary program that's

HOW TO GET A GOOD HDL READING

The nation's heart experts agree that if you're over age 20, you should be screened for both total and HDL cholesterol every five years to get the clearest picture of your heart health. (If you have other risk factors for heart disease, your doctor may recommend that you be tested more often.) But getting an accurate HDL measurement isn't easy. "The HDL test is much more difficult to perform than the test for total cholesterol," says Russell Luepker, M.D., director of the Division of Epidemiology at the University of Minnesota's School of Public Health in Minneapolis. "You can get different readings because of variations in lab methodology and biological variations, too."

How can you make sure you get the best test possible? Follow these simple guidelines.

Have your HDL tested twice within two weeks. Two tests can help correct for HDL fluctuations and variations due to lab testing, but don't wait too long between tests. "Delaying more than several weeks may affect your results because your lifestyle could change," Dr. Luepker says. "These tests need to be done in normal conditions to get the most accurate reading."

Avoid finger-stick HDL tests. They may not give the lab enough blood to work with, and there's the chance that tissue fluid may be mixed in with the sample. That could skew your test. For those reasons, it's better to have blood for your HDL test drawn from the veins in your arm.

Get tested in a hospital, clinic or doctor's office. Avoid being tested in a field setting, like a shopping mall or a mobile cholesterol screening unit. "The quality of HDL measurements in those settings has not

been demonstrated to reverse heart disease, pioneered by Dean Ornish, M.D., an assistant clinical professor of medicine at the University of California and director of

yet reached state of the art," Dr. Luepker says.

Make sure your sample's analyzed at a large laboratory. Hospitals and large clinics do enough cholesterol testing to have up-to-date equipment and staff adept at using it. And they're subject to rigid quality-control assessments, by law. While it's okay to get the blood for your test drawn in your doctor's office, don't get your sample analyzed there. The small, inexpensive desktop machines some doctors have in their offices may not yield accurate results. So ask your doctor to send your sample out to a hospital, clinic or large commercial lab.

Wait two to three hours after exercise to be tested. Or have your test before you work out. "When you exercise, you lose fluids—that tends to produce abnormal blood values for a variety of things, including HDL," Dr. Luepker says.

Watch your posture. Whether you're flat on your back or sitting upright may affect your HDL level. One position isn't necessarily better than the other—it's more important that, if you're sitting during your first test, you assume the same position for the second. That way, you eliminate fluctuations that may occur in your test results because of your posture.

Don't worry about fasting. Unless you're also getting your triglycerides checked, that is. "Eating before your blood test doesn't seem to make much difference for either total cholesterol or HDL," Dr. Luepker says. "but it can affect triglyceride levels." If you are being screened for triglycerides, too, you should abstain from food and drink (water is acceptable) for 12 to 14 hours before your test.

the Preventive Medicine Research Institute in Sausalito. According to Dr. Ornish, program participants showed significant drops in total cholesterol and LDL cholesterol, a slight reduction in HDL cholesterol and an increase in triglycerides. However, the reduction in HDL and increase in triglycerides is not likely to be harmful.

"Many experts believe that stress plays a role, but no one has done a well-controlled, large-scale trial that teaches people to relax and then measures their lipid levels and rate of heart disease," Dr. Castelli says. "Stress management may help, and it can't hurt, but if you lose weight, stop smoking, exercise and eat right, it doesn't matter what personality type you are or how much stress you're under—you can reduce your risk of heart disease substantially."

Nutrition and Health Updates

Healing Cultures

Many people have been using yogurt for years to help fight infection and stay healthy. Now new findings are finally giving the beneficial bugs in yogurt their due.

In a preliminary study, after eating yogurt containing live cultures every day for six months, 13 women with a history of vaginal yeast infections significantly cut their risk for getting new infections. The average number of infections dropped from 2.5 per woman to less than 1.

In another study, 68 people who ate two cups of yogurt with live cultures produced four times more gamma interferon in their blood than folks who ate yogurt that had been heat treated (which kills the cultures) or who avoided yogurt altogether. The increased gamma interferon—produced by disease-fighting white blood cells—suggests the bacteria may somehow boost the immune system.

"We were surprised by these results, but even more amazed that they persisted two months after the people were no longer eating the yogurt," says Georges Halpern, M.D., adjunct professor of medicine in the Department of Internal Medicine at the University of California, Davis, and author of the immunity study.

Dr. Halpern thinks the yogurt's bacteria work by stimulating parts of the immune system inside the intestinal tract. "They may also nurture a healthier environment in the intestine," he says. While these findings are very encouraging, continuing studies will be needed to confirm the results.

The words "live active cultures" seen on many yogurt containers refer to the organisms *Lactobacillus bulgaricus* and *Streptococcus thermophilus*, which turn milk into yogurt. Those were the cultures tested in Dr. Halpern's immunity study. In the vaginitis study, however, the culture at work was *Lactobacillus acidophilus*, which isn't always found in store-bought yogurt. You can check local supermarkets to see if they carry yogurt with this type of bacteria (it should say so on the container), but a better bet may be checking health-food stores. They usually carry regional brands that contain all of these healthy bugs.

Put the Lid on Cold Sores

Just because the sun comes out doesn't mean a cold sore has to follow. New research suggests that using simple sunblock on the lips may prevent sun-induced sores from sprouting.

In one study, 38 patients who had previously experienced cold sores (Type 1 herpes simplex virus) covered their lips with a sunscreen (providing a sun protection factor of 15) or a placebo ointment before they were exposed to an ultraviolet-light source. After at least three weeks, the researchers repeated the experiment using the alternate treatment for each patient. The light source was equivalent to 80 minutes of afternoon sun. The combined results showed that oral herpes developed in 71 percent of the people when they used the fake ointment, but herpes sores were completely prevented when patients used sunblock.

"Sunlight triggers roughly 25 percent of all cold sore outbreaks," says James F. Rooney, M.D., clinical virologist in the laboratory of oral medicine at the National Institutes of Health in Bethesda, Maryland. "But if used regularly, sunblock could prevent many—perhaps millions—of herpes outbreaks." This in turn may help reduce transmission of the virus, especially from parent to child.

A sunblock solution was used in the study, though Dr. Rooney thinks lip balms containing sunblock should be similarly effective. "And since sunblock can come off during eating and kissing, you should apply it once before sun exposure and then routinely thereafter to prevent inadvertent removal," he says.

Waterproof sunscreen may be even better if you're hitting the beach. You don't need to apply the sunscreen every day. But it's a good idea to use it when sun exposure is prolonged—during an outdoorsy vacation, for example, or if you're working or playing outside long enough to get a mild sunburn, he says. "Sunscreens can also help prevent skin cancer and photoaging. This study's evidence provides another reason to get people who are susceptible to cold sores to start using sunscreens," Dr. Rooney says.

Pump Up Immunity

There are a lot of things you can do to make yourself appear younger: Dye your hair, throw on ripped jeans and rock out to Bruce Springsteen. But there's one thing you can do to actually make yourself younger—not just in perception but also in reality. Get a flu vaccination.

New research suggests that the flu shot not only prevents influenza viral infections, but if taken yearly by older adults, it can also power up the immune system so it's just as potent as younger folks'. When a group of normal adults in their seventies were given a vaccine containing three strains of virus, their declining immune systems were so bolstered that they matched those of a group of young adults used for comparison.

"We found that it not only boosted responses against strains we targeted but also others not included in the vaccine," says geriatrician Janet E. McElhaney, M.D., assistant professor of medicine at the University of Alberta in Edmonton. "It would be interesting to see if these vaccines would provide an immunity boost against other illnesses."

The vaccination works by charging up your helper T-cells' memory for many different flu strains. These immune cells are left over from an original response to the virus that hit when you were younger. They still float around in the blood and still "remember" the virus, though it's a foggy recollection. But the vaccine helps jog that memory so the cells react faster when the virus shows up again. Then you won't get sick, or at least your symptoms will be much less serious.

This is not the first time a study has shown that this kind of immune reversal is possible, but it's the first to suggest that an age-related decline in the T-cell memory actually exists, says Dr. McElhaney. Because the memory recharge is only temporary, though, the vaccination should be given yearly to keep the T-cells' memory youthful.

Don't forget to get your shot early—it takes at least a few weeks before it really kicks in. And remember, the vaccine won't guard against all strains—one protective shot is no excuse to get cocky about your health.

Potassium Puts Down Blood Pressure

If your neighborhood pharmacy followed the lead of the latest research, then alongside the aisles of painkillers and greeting cards would be an abundant produce section.

Here's why: For the first time, researchers have found that boosting potassium intake may greatly slash the need for blood pressure drugs in people with hypertension.

In a study of 54 adults on antihypertension medication, 28 were placed on a high-potassium diet, which included legumes, fruits and vegetables. The remaining 26 kept to their normal diets.

After one year, 38 percent of those in the potassium group were able to stop drug therapy, compared with only 9 percent in the other group. By the end of the study, blood pressure could be controlled using less than half the amount of drugs in 81 percent of the potassium group. In the other group, only 29 percent could do the same. The high-potassium grazers also reported fewer symptoms linked to high blood pressure than the other group.

"This really shows what you can accomplish with a diet rich in potassium," says Louis Tobian, M.D., head of the High Blood Pressure Section at the University of Minnesota Hospital in Minneapolis. "Potassium seems to help make blood pressure drugs work more efficiently, so less medication is needed—until finally some people can go off medication entirely."

The dietary shift in the high-potassium group wasn't drastic, either—the study participants simply boosted their normal intake by an average of about 60 percent. They enjoyed three to six single servings of high-potassium foods, among them beans, potatoes, bananas, grapefruit, peppers and squash. The group steamed rather than boiled the legumes and vegetables to retain more of the nutrients.

This preliminary study needs to be confirmed on larger numbers of people. If you currently take antihypertension medication, don't stop taking it or start potassium supplementation without checking with your doctor.

Beans without Embarrassment

Although beans are among the healthiest foods you can eat, they have an unfortunate habit of talking back. There is one product, however, that will allow you to enjoy your bowl of beans without enduring their noisy and sometimes painful epilogue.

In one study, 38 adults were fed a bowl of refried black beans. Those with high levels of hydrogen (H_2) in their breath (which corresponds to gas levels) after the first meal went on to eat more beans, this time with a substance called alpha-galactosidase sprinkled on top. This naturally derived enzyme is contained in a product called Beano.

With successive additions of the enzyme (5, 10 and 70 drops), their peak H_2 responses dropped accordingly. Most gaseous symptoms also improved significantly.

"The enzyme works by breaking down indigestible sugars in the beans while they're still in the stomach," says bean expert Joseph Maga, Ph.D., director of the Food Research and Development Center at Colorado State University in Fort Collins. "These sugars then end up being absorbed into the bloodstream, where they can't cause any more trouble."

If the sugars aren't caught by the enzyme, they're used by bacteria as food. This in turn causes gas, gas pain and—depending on where you are—some embarrassment.

To use Beano, just add it to your first bite of food. The drops don't affect the taste of the food and won't add any additional calories to the meal. And since extreme heat destroys the gas-stopping enzyme, Beano will not be effective if used while cooking.

The manufacturers claim Beano also works on cabbage, oats, soy foods and other healthy but gas-producing foods, although those weren't tested in this study.

People with diabetes, mold- and penicillin-sensitive people and galactosemics shouldn't use Beano without first checking with their doctor. Beano is available nationwide at most supermarkets and pharmacies.

Giving the Lie to Heartburn

Dinner and dessert are history—now you're heading for the couch to assume the snooze position.

Wait! Don't lie on your right side, lie on your left. When it comes to avoiding heartburn, left may actually be right.

In one study, 20 people sat down for a fatty meal (61 percent of calories from fat) in order to create heartburn. Then they went horizontal for a four-hour nap. Total minutes of heartburn were measured. Researchers, and the snoozers, found that the total amount of heartburn was greater for those lying on the right versus the left side.

The reasoning behind a left-side lie is simple. "The stomach is lower when you're lying on your left side," says William Ruderman, M.D., chairman of gastroenterology at the Cleveland Clinic–Florida in Fort Lauderdale. "So if you lie on your left, stomach acid (the instigator of heartburn) pools and won't go anywhere." If you lie on the right side, though, the acid has to move somewhere, and it usually makes a beeline toward your esophagus, where it irritates the tender lining and so causes heartburn.

Try these tips as your first line of attack.

■ With blocks or books, elevate the head of the bed (or sofa) four to six inches. "That lets gravity keep the stomach acid where it belongs," says Dr. Ruderman.

■ Take a postprandial stroll. "Sit down after eating and you'll soon give way to a slump—and suddenly you're snoozing," says Dr. Ruderman. "Take a relaxed, not fast, walk to help let the food pass," he says.

■ Take a look, too, at the food to see if there's a repeat offender in your diet. Spicy or acidic foods, as well as a high-fat diet, can cause heartburn. Keeping antacid tablets nearby may also help.

Practice Your High C

You can't turn back time. But there's one nutrient that may allow you to get your hands on more of it. Research suggests that people who get high levels of vitamin C every day may live longer by reducing their heart disease risk.

In a ten-year study of 11,348 adults, men in the group that had the highest intake of vitamin C had a 41 percent lower death rate during that period compared with men taking in less than 50 milligrams naturally. The high-intake group averaged 300 milligrams per day (at least 50 milligrams from food, plus regular use of supplements, mostly multivitamins).

In addition, men in the high-C group were 45 percent less likely to die of heart disease than men in the low-intake group. Women in the high-intake group experienced a 10 percent lower overall death rate and a 25 percent lower heart disease death rate than the low-intake group.

"I've been studying vitamin C for some time, but I didn't expect to see such a large effect," says James Enstrom, Ph.D., an epidemiologist from the University of California, Los Angeles. In fact, Dr. Enstrom tried to control for other lifestyle factors and behaviors that may have also played a role in increasing life span. Vitamin C still climbed above the pack. "This is an area that really needs to be looked at more," he adds.

"In the last 20 years, the death rate from heart disease has been cut in half," he says. "Over that same period, the use of vitamin C has increased. This study suggests a strong connection between these two events."

The key to vitamin C may be in its antioxidant properties—blocking the activity of highly unstable molecules of oxygen that damage cells and may promote heart disease. Although vitamin C did display its own independent effect, its use may also be indicative of other beneficial lifestyle behaviors that promote a longer life. "Someone who takes vitamin C every day may also practice other healthy habits," says Dr. Enstrom.

Lower Pressure, More Pleasure

We've reported many times that lowering blood pressure naturally—by exercising, eating well and reducing stress—is often just as effective as blood pressure drugs in treating hypertension. That's good news for men, since blood pressure drugs often take a tremendous toll on their sex life.

But here's even better news: Lowering blood pressure naturally doesn't just preserve your sex life—it boosts it!

In a study, researchers divided 79 hypertensive men into three groups: One group embarked on the nondrug treatment, while the remaining men either received the common antihypertensive drug propranolol or took a placebo pill.

The research confirmed that lifestyle changes do indeed improve blood pressure. But the really exciting news was that lowering blood pressure alone, without drugs, had a positive impact on sexual arousal and pleasure.

"This is the first time we've shown that lowering blood pressure by lifestyle changes in and of itself improves sex life, compared with those men with high blood pressure who did nothing to lower it," says John B. Kostis, M.D., chairman of the Department of Medicine at the University of Medicine and Dentistry of New Jersey, Robert Wood Johnson Medical School, in New Brunswick.

That amazing finding should be enough to get any hypertensive man (and his partner) thinking about getting his pressure down. But there's more: The men's body weight dropped, as did total and LDL cholesterol (the harmful kind).

These improved lovers embarked on numerous heart-healthy changes, such as cutting down on fat, salt and alcohol, walking and riding bikes for exercise and using relaxation techniques to tackle stress.

"This strengthens the idea that nondrug approaches to high blood pressure should be the first road taken," says Dr. Kostis. Do not, of course, adjust your medication without first talking to your doctor.

189
■

Wheat Whips Cholesterol

Oat bran isn't the only high-fiber food that's been found to lower cholesterol. In one study, 19 adults with high cholesterol received 20 grams a day of raw wheat germ or partially defatted wheat germ for 4 weeks. The amounts were then kicked up to 30 grams a day for 14 weeks. After these 14 weeks, those getting the raw wheat germ had a drop in cholesterol of 7.2 percent—representing a potential 15 percent decrease in coronary heart disease.

The raw wheat germ also was associated with a drop in LDL cholesterol of 15.4 percent, an 11.3 percent drop in triglycerides and a decrease in another possible heart risk factor called the "apo B:apo A1 ratio." Total HDL cholesterol didn't vary. The other wheat germ formulation appeared to have an effect at four weeks but tapered off by the end of the study. The study needs to be repeated with a larger group of people to confirm these results.

"It's still not clearly understood, but the vitamin E substance in the wheat germ oil (called tocotrienol) may help prevent coronary disease by blocking cholesterol synthesis in the liver," speculates Michael H. Davidson, M.D., medical director at St. Luke's Medical Center in Chicago. This antioxidant substance potentially prevents healthy LDL cholesterol particles from becoming oxidized and going rancid. "If they go rancid, it's thought they can be incorporated faster into artery walls, clogging up the vessels and leading to heart disease," he says.

The study participants didn't need much wheat germ to help their lipid levels. The amount used was roughly equal to ¼ cup—spoonfuls easily slipped into a normal diet. "Use it in meat loaf or lean ground meat, or sprinkle it on cereal," says Dr. Davidson.

In this study, only the effect of wheat germ was under scrutiny. The fat content of the diet—which was high—wasn't tampered with. "If the benefit of wheat germ is confirmed," Dr. Davidson says, "then perhaps you can anticipate an additional benefit by reducing fat intake along with adding wheat germ to your diet."

Head-to-Heart Protection

The heart and the eyes. According to new research, both of these might benefit from vitamin E.

A small pilot study suggests the nutrient may help the ticker by slowing atherosclerosis. Two groups of 12 normal men were given either 800 international units per day of vitamin E or a placebo for 12 weeks. In men getting vitamin E, LDL cholesterol was 50 percent less likely to undergo oxidation. That's a process in which free-radical oxygen molecules cause those cholesterol particles to turn rancid. Researchers speculate that this in turn could lead to clogged arteries.

"The dose was much higher than the Recommended Dietary Allowance (RDA)—but this is a whole new ball game," says Ishwarlal Jialal, M.D., Ph.D., associate professor of internal medicine and clinical nutrition at the University of Texas Southwestern Medical Center in Dallas. "The RDA pertains to deficiency problems—we're talking about a different potential function in decreasing heart attack risk."

Vitamin E has also been linked to a lower risk of one of the most common cataract formations, called a nuclear cataract. "The risk for this cataract was roughly cut in half in people who had the highest blood levels of vitamin E," says Susan Vitale, assistant professor of ophthalmology at Johns Hopkins University in Baltimore, commenting on a study involving 832 people.

The nutrient, she believes, may help by shielding the lens against oxidative damage, which may be caused by factors such as cigarette smoking. Talk to your doctor if you're considering taking E in large doses, since it may interact with other medications.

Future Youth

Uncle Ned says he can't do this and he can't do that. When you ask him why, he shrugs and says, "I'm just getting older." If Uncle Ned doesn't watch out, that excuse may get the best of him.

A study suggests that older adults who attribute their health status to getting older have a 78 percent greater risk of dying earlier than those who don't use aging as an excuse.

Researchers looked at a group of 1,391 adults aged 70 and older who experienced difficulties in daily functions and asked them why their problems occurred. Those who blamed their problems on aging tended to die sooner than those who could give specific, nonaging reasons for their problem.

"Once you say a problem is due to old age, you may resign yourself to thinking it isn't treatable and delay seeking care," says William Rakowski, Ph.D., of the Center for Gerontology and Health Care Research at Brown University in Providence, Rhode Island. "You've given up in a way."

We often talk about prevention in terms of the physical—that getting plenty of exercise and sticking to a healthy diet may help you live longer. But prevention is mental, too. "We can't promise optimism will actually make you live longer," says Dr. Rakowski. "But the alternative of giving up, this study suggests, may set you up for adverse health in the long run." What's his advice? "Keep fighting."

Fish Oil Keeps Arteries in the Swim

The trouble with opening blocked coronary arteries with balloon angioplasty is that all too often they close again, usually within six months after the operation. Heart specialists have been searching for ways to keep arteries clear longer. The answer, it appears, may be fish oil.

In one study, doctors at Laval University and the Quebec Heart Institute in Canada put half the people on a regimen of 15 fish-oil capsules a day for three weeks before they underwent angioplasty and for six months afterward. The other half got olive oil capsules.

All the patients underwent an angiogram six months after the angioplasty. The results were measured by computer analysis. Using this very objective standard, the heart specialists found that the people who had taken fish-oil capsules had significantly less reblockage—22 to 35 percent—compared with 40 to 53 percent in people who took olive oil (similar to what happens to angioplasty patients who make no dietary changes after the procedure).

"Our results show that we are able to decrease the rate of restenosis (reblockage) after angioplasty by one-third with fish-oil supplements," says Louis Roy, M.D., one of the directors of the study. "So far, nothing else has been shown to be as effective."

What's more, when they asked patients about their typical diets, the doctors found that people eating more than one gram per week of omega-3 fatty acids (about the amount in 7½ ounces of seafood) had less reblockage. So Dr. Roy thinks it's possible that just substituting fish for meat several times a week may eventually be shown to keep arteries open.

"It may be that there is something besides the oil in fish that hasn't been identified yet that also may be active in preventing restenosis. So we may find that patients can just eat fish three times a week to maintain the effects of the angioplasty."

193

Exercise Your Energy

A quick fix of sugary, fatty snacks or a cigarette may jump-start your mood at a down moment. But as that pick-me-up quickly wears off, the unhealthy consequences remain. Instead of that harmful route, take another path—with a few minutes of walking.

A group of 16 addicted smokers and 18 regular snackers kept track of their moods and urges while either taking regular ten-minute brisk walks during the study or remaining inactive. Researchers found that the short, brisk jaunts were enough to cream the cravings—and have a positive effect on mood. Compared with those who remained inactive, the walkers were able to go longer between smokes or a snack.

"Moderate exercise clearly reduced the urge for these unhealthy substances," says study author Robert E. Thayer, Ph.D., of California State University, in Long Beach, author of *Biopsychology of Mood and Arousal*. "When people look for something to pick up their moods, they may be able to substitute a walk for that cupcake or cigarette."

Previous research has suggested a biochemical basis for this mood-boosting effect—that exercise stimulates production of chemicals in the brain that help make us feel better. Dr. Thayer, though, thinks there's a lot more to it than that. "Exercise stimulates not just the brain but a whole number of different systems in the body, as well. It simultaneously acts upon our cardiovascular system, our glands, our breathing and more."

Since people use all sorts of substances to manipulate their moods, this research points out healthier ways to go about it. "Of course, this is nothing new to someone who exercises regularly," says Dr. Thayer. "They already know exercise is the magic elixir—decreasing appetite and improving one's mood." A short burst of exercise can do this, but long-term benefits of regular exercise itself—weight loss and a healthier heart—shouldn't hurt in keeping your spirits high, either.

Walk Off Arthritis

If your knees ache due to osteoarthritis, and you ask your doctor about walking, you'll hear one of two things: Yes, you can walk to boost your health and to ease arthritic symptoms; or no, you shouldn't walk—the pain may get worse.

Up until now, doctors haven't been sure what to tell patients with painful knees. But one study, conducted at the Hospital for Special Surgery and Columbia University in New York City and funded by the Arthritis Foundation, may clear up the confusion.

In this study of 102 people with osteoarthritis of the knee, patient education and a supervised walking program both improved the ability of patients to walk and decreased the amount of pain they felt. Control patients who didn't walk experienced a 55-foot decrease in their ability to walk. The walkers increased their ability to walk by nearly 230 feet. They also felt 27 percent less pain after the eight-week program and used less medication than nonwalkers.

The walkers spent three days a week walking indoors for 30 minutes. (Some strengthening and stretching exercises were carried out before each trek.) About an hour was spent educating them on the benefits of exercise. They were told about proper techniques, shoes and clothing.

For tips on exercising with arthritis, call the Arthritis Foundation at (800) 283-7800. In Canada, contact the Arthritis Society, National Communications Office, 250 Bloor St. E., Suite 401, Toronto, ON M4W 3P2 (a self-addressed, stamped envelope would be appreciated). If you have severe hip, knee or ankle problems, see your doctor before starting a walking program.

Drink In the Sunshine

A dark winter can do more than chill the bones—it can drain them, too. During those cold months, the sun, which turns our skin on to produce bone-building vitamin D, takes some time off. Studies have suggested that this seasonal variation slows vitamin D production and so leads to harmful bone loss.

For the first time, researchers have looked closely to see if they can protect against this wintry bone drain by giving vitamin D supplements.

They gave 249 healthy postmenopausal women either 400 international units of vitamin D (the amount added to a quart of milk) or a placebo daily for one year. Spine and whole-body bone scans were done at different times during the study. In the placebo group, spinal bone density increased in the summer and fall months and decreased in the winter to spring months. In other words, the group experienced no net change in bone.

Women treated with vitamin D supplements, on the other hand, had similar increases in spinal density in the first period but less loss in the winter months. They experienced a significant overall benefit when the year was up.

"A substantial body of evidence suggests this bone fluctuation will occur year in and year out," says Bess Dawson-Hughes, M.D., from the USDA Human Nutrition Research Center on Aging at Tufts University in Boston. "Since vitamin D insufficiency can contribute to this bone loss, it may be appropriate to bring it up to healthy levels with diet or supplementation."

Most of us can get enough vitamin D by drinking a quart of D-fortified milk daily. If you can't drink that much milk and decide to take a vitamin D supplement, take no more than 400 international units daily. Researchers urge you to use caution in taking amounts higher than that.

As part of a variation on this study, both the vitamin D and the placebo groups were taking calcium supplements. "We suspect that the bone loss would have been even worse had they not been taking the calcium as well," says Dr. Dawson-Hughes.

Fabulous Everyday Recipes

22 This Fowl Is First-Rate Fare

Four great ways to prepare chicken.

Not so long ago, chicken was a special-occasion food, reserved for Sunday dinners or noteworthy celebrations. Today it's everyday fare, making frequent weekday appearances on tables nationwide. In the past four years alone, poultry consumption has risen ten pounds per person to reach an all-time yearly high of almost 70 pounds!

Why? Consumers perceive poultry as a lean and healthy source of protein. And the facts bear them out. A 3½-ounce serving of roasted chicken breast, for example, has only 3.6 grams of fat and 165 calories. Figures for leg meat are a little higher: 8.4 grams of fat and 191 calories. Both are lower than many cuts of red meat.

A second aspect of chicken's popularity is its supreme versatility. You can dress it up, dress it down and serve it seven days a week without having the same dish twice.

Every cut of chicken has its own distinct flavor and texture. Because chickens do a lot of standing around and little flying, they have white, mild-flavored, tender breast meat. Their legs get much more exercise and turn out darker and firmer, with a stronger, gamier flavor. By using the right cooking method, the white meat will be flavorful and juicy and the dark meat will be deliciously tender.

The simplest way to prepare chicken is to roast it. Roast chicken is the quintessential homestyle dish, far better when made there than in a restaurant—although many four-star chefs are judged by their ability to make this simple dish.

But all too often, restaurant roast chicken has been cooked ahead. And precooked meats lose precious juices as they sit waiting to be ordered. At home, you have a luxury that's really rare in restaurants: time enough to prepare food to order and serve it perfectly done. Succulent, savory roast chicken every time will be your reward when you try the following technique.

Roasting Basics

Here's one of the best ways to roast a chicken. For a variation, try the garlic and rosemary version at the end of the basic recipe. It will fill your kitchen with the smell of caramelized garlic and resinous rosemary.

■ Start with a whole chicken that weighs three to five pounds. Rinse with cold water and pat dry with paper towels. Season inside and out with plenty of black pepper and, if desired, a small amount of kosher salt.

■ Preheat the oven to 400°F.

■ A chicken that is roasted at a high temperature will have a much deeper and richer flavor because of the caramelization of its juices. It will, however, tend to shrink more than a bird done at a lower temperature.

■ To obtain the best color and flavor, use a dark-colored steel, cast-iron or enameled pan just big enough to hold the bird. A dark pan absorbs rather than reflects the heat, and metal conducts the heat much better than glass or ceramic. An important point: Because chicken does not brown as much in a glass or ceramic pan, you risk overcooking it and drying out the white meat if you let appearance alone be your guide to doneness.

■ Place the chicken, breast side up, in the pan on a roasting rack and roast it for 1 to 1¼ hours. Surprisingly, the difference in cooking time between a three-pound and a five-pound bird is only about 15 minutes. After the first 30 minutes of roasting, carefully pour off and discard any excess fat that has dripped into the pan. Repeat this procedure during the last 15 minutes of cooking.

■ Test for doneness by piercing the inner thigh, since this is the part that takes the longest to cook. The juices that run out should be clear rather than pink. Remove the chicken from the pan and place it on a heated serving dish.

■ If you'd like, you may deglaze the pan. Pour off any fat and add about two cups of liquid, such as defatted chicken stock, vegetable stock, cider or water spiked with a little fruit vinegar. Place the pan (make sure it's stovetop safe) directly on a burner and bring the liquid to a boil. Turn down the heat and simmer about ten minutes, scraping up the browned bits by using a wooden spoon. Pour the liquid through a sieve, if desired, to remove any solid particles.

■ Meanwhile, remove the skin from the bird. Carve the chicken into serving portions. Serve with the deglazing juices, if desired.

Here's a variation that combines the traditional French method using 40 cloves of garlic with the Italian touch of tucking rosemary sprigs under the skin.

■ Before you season the chicken with pepper and salt, carefully separate the skin from the flesh over the breast side. Insert a handful of rosemary leaves under the skin.

■ Separate two whole heads of garlic into individual cloves and peel. Fill the cavity with the garlic. Throw in a handful of rosemary sprigs. Season the bird as directed.

■ Roast the chicken for about 45 minutes. Pour off any fat from the pan. Using a wooden spoon, remove the garlic cloves from inside the chicken. Scatter them around the chicken in the roasting pan. Return the pan to the oven and finish the recipe. Be sure to deglaze the pan to take advantage of all the flavor from the roasted garlic.

Other Cooking Methods

Other recipes that are included here use the techniques of poaching, stewing and pan-roasting. With these healthy, tasty recipes, you can dress up a chicken dinner and never be bored. Serve a magnificent roast bird for company, cook a skillet dish for a casual meal or sample a marinade at an outdoor grilling party.

Poulet Niçoise

- 1 bunch fresh basil, leaves only
- 8 chicken thighs, skinned, with all visible fat removed
- ½ cup unbleached flour
- ¾ cup defatted chicken stock
- 1 red onion, thinly sliced
- 6–8 cloves garlic, peeled and sliced
  - Pinch of ground cloves
  - Juice and grated rind of 1 orange
  - Pinch of saffron (optional)
- 10 tiny black olives, pitted and halved
- 1 pint ripe cherry tomatoes, halved
  - Ground black pepper
- 4 cups hot cooked couscous

Neatly stack the basil leaves on top of each other. Roll up the stack to resemble a cigar. Thinly slice the leaves crosswise using a sharp knife; set aside.

Dredge the chicken in flour to coat lightly; knock off excess flour. In a 10" or 12" heavy frying pan (preferably cast-iron) over medium-high heat, warm ¼ cup of the stock. Add the chicken in a single layer. Cook until browned on both sides. Remove and set aside.

Add the onion, garlic and cloves. Sauté for a few minutes to soften the onion; do not let the garlic burn.

Add the orange juice and rind, saffron, olives and the remaining ½ cup stock. Mix well. Return the chicken to the pan. Bring the liquid to a boil.

Reduce the heat to medium. Simmer for 20 minutes. Add the cherry tomatoes, black pepper and reserved basil. Simmer for 10 minutes, or until the chicken is cooked through. Serve with the couscous.

Serves 4

Per serving: 495 calories, 9.6 grams fat (17% of calories), 10.8 grams dietary fiber, 37.8 grams protein, 65.5 grams carbohydrate, 114 milligrams cholesterol, 241 milligrams sodium. Also a very good source of niacin, pantothenic acid, vitamin B_6 and vitamin C.

Chicken-in-a-Pot with Root Vegetables

16 chicken thighs, skinned, with all visible fat removed
2 quarts defatted chicken stock
½ pound carrots, peeled and cut into chunks
1 large turnip, peeled and cut into chunks
1 large celery root, peeled and cut into chunks
1 small butternut squash, peeled, seeded and diced
2 leeks, sliced into rings and washed thoroughly
1 thin loaf (baguette) sourdough, Italian or French bread
2 cloves garlic, halved
2 tablespoons olive oil
¼ cup grated Asiago or Parmesan cheese
½ bunch dill, chopped

Place the chicken in a 4-quart or larger pot. Add the stock. Bring to a boil. Simmer for 45 minutes, or until the chicken is cooked through. Remove the chicken, place on a plate, cover and refrigerate. Leave the stock in the pot or pour it into a large bowl. Refrigerate overnight. The next day, remove the hardened fat from the surface and discard it.

Return the defatted stock to the pot. Add the carrots, turnips, celery root, squash and leeks. Bring to a boil. Simmer for 15 minutes. Add the reserved chicken. Simmer for 10 minutes longer.

Meanwhile, split the bread in half lengthwise. Rub the interior with the garlic. Drizzle lightly with the oil. Sprinkle with the cheese. Re-form the loaf. Wrap it in foil and bake at 400° for 15 minutes. Cut into slices.

To serve the soup, place 2 thighs in the bottom of each deep soup bowl. Ladle vegetables and stock into the bowl. Sprinkle with the dill and serve with the bread.

Serves 8

Per serving: 437 calories, 11.4 grams fat (24% of calories), 6 grams dietary fiber, 35.9 grams protein, 46.8 grams carbohydrate, 116 milligrams cholesterol, 530 milligrams sodium. Also a very good source of niacin, vitamin A, vitamin C, vitamin B_6 and potassium.

202

Skillet-Roasted Chicken

1 small (2–2½ pounds) broiler or fryer chicken
4 ounces shiitake mushrooms, stems
   removed and caps quartered
4 ounces white mushrooms, quartered
8 scallions, cut into 1" lengths
½ cup defatted chicken stock
¼ cup lemon juice
½ bunch fresh Italian parsley, leaves only
½ bunch fresh tarragon, leaves only
   Ground black pepper, to taste
2 cups hot cooked rice

Split the chicken in half lengthwise and remove the backbone. Cut each piece in half crosswise. Cut 2 to 3 slashes in each thigh.

Over medium-high heat, heat a 10" or 12" well-seasoned cast-iron frying pan until quite hot, about 5 minutes. Place the chicken, skin side down, in the pan. Cover the pieces with a second frying pan and a foil-wrapped brick to weigh them down.

Reduce the heat to medium. Cook for about 15 minutes. Flip the pieces, weigh them down again and cook for another 15 minutes. Check to see if the chicken is cooked through by piercing the thighs in the thickest part; the juices that run out should be clear, not pink.

Remove the pieces from the pan. Peel off and discard the skin. Place the chicken on a plate and keep it warm.

Wipe the main frying pan with paper towels. Add the mushrooms. Sauté for about 4 minutes. Add the scallions; cook for 1 to 2 minutes. Add the stock, lemon juice, parsley, tarragon and pepper. Simmer for about 5 minutes, or until the liquid has reduced and is syrupy.

Pour the sauce over the chicken. Serve with the rice.

Serves 4

Per serving: 398 calories, 9.3 grams fat (21% of calories), 2.1 grams dietary fiber, 38 grams protein, 39.8 grams carbohydrate, 101 milligrams cholesterol, 116 milligrams sodium. Also a very good source of niacin, vitamin B_6 and selenium.

23

Beef Up with Beans

High in fiber, protein and complex carbohydrates, legumes pack a cholesterol-pounding punch.

Lentils were King Tut's favorite food. Well, probably not. But they could have been. These little legumes are among the world's oldest domesticated crops, dating back a good 10,000 years. The same goes for their cousins, the split peas. Regardless of how much ancient Egyptian royalty actually relished them, these foods (which belong to the legume family, along with beans) deserve a princely place in your diet.

We've known for some time now that beans, lentils and peas are much more than "poor-man's meat." They're rich in protein and hunger-appeasing complex carbohydrates. What's more, they're low in fat and sodium and have no cholesterol. Better still, they can help you lower your cholesterol. Studies done by James W. Anderson, M.D., professor of medicine and clinical nutrition at the University of Kentucky College of Medicine, have borne this out.

Legumes contain lots of soluble fiber. And it's this fiber that has such cholesterol-pounding potential, according to Dr. Anderson.

In one study, Dr. Anderson gave people with dangerously high cholesterol levels (about 260) 1½ cups of cooked beans a day for three weeks. The results of the study were dramatic: Total cholesterol fell an average of 60 points. This was similar to the effect of oat bran, which also caused large decreases, says Dr. Anderson.

Naturally, your results on a legume-intensive diet could vary, depending on lots of individual factors, such as your current cholesterol level. "People with readings over 250 show better results than those with levels in the low 200s," says Dr. Anderson. Still, there's little reason not to make legumes a prominent part of your diet.

Bean Power in a Flash

Well, one reason might be that you may think that they take too long to prepare. Indeed, dried beans do require a lot of prep time. First you need to soak them for several hours, then cook them for a few more. All of which brings us back to lentils and split peas. These legumes require no soaking whatsoever, so you don't have to plan ahead. And they cook up in a mere fraction of the time other dried beans demand.

Further, says Dr. Anderson, "although split peas and lentils are a little lower in fiber than the beans we used in our study, they should still have a good cholesterol-lowering effect."

Lentils come in shades of green, brown and reddish-orange. Split peas are available in green and yellow. That means you've got plenty of versatility—and all your meals won't look alike. To use these legumes, simply pour them into a bowl and rinse with cold water. Pick out any dark or discolored pieces, then drain in a colander. Cook split peas and lentils in water or stock until just the right texture for your recipe. Here are some guidelines from the USA Dry Pea and Lentil Council: For al dente split peas to toss with pasta or to use in salads, 20 to 25 minutes will do it. For soups or purees, increase the time to 30 to 45 minutes. Green and brown lentils take about 15 to 20 minutes on the stove. And orange ones cook even faster: they're ready in 5 to 10 minutes.

If the only way you've ever eaten split peas and lentils is in a thick, hambone-flavored soup, you'll be pleased to know there are lots of other wonderful uses for these legumes. They're terrific in salads, casseroles, dips, pilafs, stuffings and more. Talented cookbook author Marie Simmons has created a half dozen easy, tempting recipes to help you make split peas and lentils a regular part of your diet.

Among them are Rice and Lentil Patties, a meaty alternative to burgers, with considerably less fat. Lentil and Chicory Vinaigrette is a hearty, warm salad that can be on the table in about 25 minutes. Yellow Split-Pea Dip is an easy dish that can be prepared ahead and served as a party appetizer or even a snack. Two deliciously different combos are Lentils with Curried Vegetables and Pasta with Split Peas in Spicy Tomato Sauce. And for a new spin on split-pea soup, try Split-Pea and Spinach Soup with Garlic Yogurt, which you can also make ahead and reheat.

So do something nice for your cholesterol. Invite lentils and split peas for dinner—often!

Rice and Lentil Patties with Curried Tomato Sauce

Curried Tomato Sauce
1 teaspoon olive oil
2 tablespoons finely chopped onions
1 teaspoon finely chopped fresh ginger
½ teaspoon minced garlic
2 teaspoons curry powder
½ teaspoon ground cumin
    Pinch of ground red pepper
1 can (14 ounces) whole tomatoes with juice, coarsely chopped
1 tablespoon finely chopped fresh coriander

Rice and Lentil Patties
1 cup cooked medium- or short-grain white rice, at room temperature (see Note)
1 cup cooked green lentils, at room temperature (see Note)
1 tablespoon olive oil
1 cup finely chopped onions
1 tablespoon finely chopped hot green chili peppers (wear plastic gloves when handling)
1 clove garlic, minced
1 teaspoon cumin seeds
1 egg white, beaten until frothy

To make the curried tomato sauce: In a large no-stick frying pan over medium heat, warm the oil. Add the onions, ginger and garlic. Cook, stirring constantly, for 5 minutes. Add the curry powder, cumin and red pepper; stir for 1 minute.

Add the tomatoes and bring to a boil. Cook, stirring often and breaking up the tomatoes with the side of the spoon, until the mixture is reduced by half. Transfer to a 1-quart saucepan and keep warm over low heat. (Or refrigerate until needed; reheat before serving.) Stir in the coriander just before serving.

To make the rice and lentil patties: In a large bowl, mix the rice and lentils. Set aside.

In a large no-stick frying pan over medium-low heat, warm 2 teaspoons of the oil. Add the onions and cook, stirring often, for 10 minutes, or until the onions brown. Add the chili peppers, garlic and cumin. Cook, stirring, for 2 minutes. Add to the lentil mixture. Add the egg white and mix well.

Wet your hands with cold water and form about ¼ cup of the mixture into a firm patty about 2½" in diameter. Place on a tray lined with wax paper. Repeat with the remaining mixture to make 8 patties.

Wipe out the frying pan. Add the remaining 1 teaspoon oil and warm over medium heat. Working in batches, if necessary, brown the patties on both sides (about 5 minutes per side). Serve with the tomato sauce.

Serves 4

Note: To get 1 cup of cooked rice, start with 1¼ cups boiling water and ⅓ cup white rice. Cook for about 20 minutes, or until the rice is tender and all liquid has been absorbed; cool to room temperature. To get 1 cup cooked lentils, start with 1 quart water and ⅓ cup lentils. Cook for about 25 minutes, or until the lentils are tender; drain and cool to room temperature.

Per serving: 199 calories, 5.4 grams fat (24% of calories), 3.8 grams dietary fiber, 8 grams protein, 31.2 grams carbohydrate, no cholesterol, 212 milligrams sodium. Also a very good source of folate.

Lentil and Chicory Vinaigrette

2 quarts water
1⅓ cups green lentils, sorted and rinsed
1 bay leaf
2 sprigs celery leaves
1 carrot
2 onions
3 cloves garlic
2 tablespoons olive oil
2 ounces smoked turkey breast, cut into 1¼" slivers
1 pound chicory, trimmed and cut into 1½" pieces
¼ cup defatted chicken stock
1 tablespoon red wine vinegar
⅛ teaspoon ground black pepper

In a 3-quart saucepan, combine the water, lentils, bay leaf, celery leaves, carrot, 1 onion and 1 clove garlic. Bring to a boil over high heat. Reduce the heat to medium and simmer for 20 minutes, or until the lentils are tender. Drain. Return the lentils to the pan; discard the bay leaf, celery, onion and garlic. Thinly slice the carrot, add to the pan and set aside, off the heat.

Meanwhile, in a large no-stick frying pan over medium heat, warm 1 tablespoon of the oil. Thinly slice the remaining onion and add to the pan. Cook, stirring often, for 10 minutes, or until golden.

Thinly slice the remaining 2 cloves garlic. Add to the pan. Stir in the turkey breast; sauté for 2 minutes. Add the chicory, reserved lentil mixture and stock.

Cover and cook, stirring occasionally, for 15 minutes, or until the greens are soft. (If the mixture becomes too dry, add a little more stock or some water.) Remove from the heat and let stand, covered, for 10 minutes.

Drizzle with the vinegar, pepper and the remaining 1 tablespoon oil. Toss well to combine.

Serves 4

Per serving: 327 calories, 8.4 grams fat (23% of calories), 10.6 grams dietary fiber, 22.5 grams protein, 44.3 grams carbohydrate, 6 milligrams cholesterol, 152 milligrams sodium. Also a very good source of folate, vitamin A, vitamin C, potassium and iron.

Yellow Split-Pea Dip

¼ cup finely chopped yellow onions
2 teaspoons finely chopped fresh ginger
2 cloves garlic, minced
5 teaspoons olive oil
2 teaspoons curry powder
1 teaspoon ground cumin
½ teaspoon turmeric
1 cup yellow split peas, sorted and rinsed
4 cups water or defatted chicken stock (or a mixture)
2 tablespoons lemon juice
1 teaspoon grated lemon rind
2 tablespoons finely chopped red onions
   Pinch of ground red pepper
¼ teaspoon dried oregano

In a 2-quart saucepan over low heat, sauté the yellow onions, ginger and half of the garlic in 1 teaspoon of the oil for 3 minutes, or until the onions are tender. Stir in the curry powder, cumin and turmeric.

Add the split peas and water or stock. Increase the heat to medium-high and bring to a boil. Reduce the heat to low, cover and cook for 1¼ hours, or until the split peas are very soft and most of the liquid has been absorbed. Drain off any remaining liquid.

Transfer to a large bowl and chill for several hours or overnight. Spoon the mixture (it will be very stiff) into a food processor. Add 1½ teaspoons of the remaining oil, 1 tablespoon of the lemon juice and the lemon rind. Process until smooth, creamy and light in color.

Transfer the mixture to a shallow serving bowl and spread evenly. Sprinkle with the red onions and pepper.

In a cup, whisk together the remaining 2½ teaspoons oil and the remaining 1 tablespoon lemon juice. Add the oregano and remaining garlic; mix well. Just before serving, drizzle over the dip.

Serves 8

Per serving: 117 calories, 3.3 grams fat (25% of calories), 2.1 grams dietary fiber, 6.3 grams protein, 16.7 grams carbohydrate, no cholesterol, 9 milligrams sodium.

Lentils with Curried Vegetables

1 tablespoon olive oil
2 onions, quartered
½ cup diagonally sliced carrots
½ cup diagonally sliced celery
3 cloves garlic, coarsely chopped
1 tablespoon curry powder
1 teaspoon ground cumin
¼ teaspoon turmeric
2 cups defatted chicken stock
1 cup brown lentils, sorted and rinsed
1 sweet potato, peeled and cubed
1 thin slice fresh ginger
1 bay leaf
1 cardamom pod
1 cup chopped green beans (½" pieces)
½ cup peas
1 cup low-fat yogurt, at room temperature

In a large no-stick frying pan over medium heat, warm the oil. Add the onions, carrots and celery. Cook, stirring often, for 10 minutes, or until golden. Add the garlic and cook for 3 minutes.

Reduce the heat to low and stir in the curry powder, cumin and turmeric. Add the stock, lentils, sweet potatoes, ginger, bay leaf and cardamom. Increase the heat to medium-high and bring to a boil.

Cover and reduce the heat to low. Cook, stirring occasionally, for 20 minutes, or until the lentils are almost tender. (If the mixture becomes too dry, add a little additional stock or some water.)

Add the green beans; cover and cook for 5 minutes. Add the peas; cover and cook for 5 minutes. Remove from the heat; discard the bay leaf and cardamom. Allow the mixture to cool for approximately 5 minutes.

Place the yogurt in a large serving bowl. Gradually stir in the warm vegetable mixture.

Serves 4

Per serving: 353 calories, 6.2 grams fat (16% of calories), 8.1 grams dietary fiber, 20.7 grams protein, 57.4

grams carbohydrate, 4 milligrams cholesterol, 122 milligrams sodium. Also a very good source of folate, vitamin A, vitamin C, potassium and iron.

Pasta with Split Peas in Spicy Tomato Sauce

3 cups water
½ cup green split peas, sorted and rinsed
1 tablespoon minced garlic
½ teaspoon red-pepper flakes
2 tablespoons olive oil
1 can (28 ounces) plum tomatoes with juice
1 bay leaf
2 cups macaroni or ditalini
2 tablespoons grated Parmesan cheese

In a 2-quart saucepan over high heat, bring the water to a boil. Add the split peas. Reduce the heat to medium-low and cook, stirring occasionally, for 1¼ hours, or until the peas are tender but not mushy. Drain and set aside.

In a large no-stick frying pan over medium-low heat, cook the garlic and red-pepper flakes in the oil until the garlic starts to sizzle. Reduce the heat to low and cook for 5 minutes; do not brown the garlic.

Stir in the tomatoes and bay leaf. Increase the heat to medium-high and bring to a boil. Then reduce the heat to medium-low and simmer for 15 minutes, or until the sauce is somewhat reduced and thickened. Discard the bay leaf.

Cook the pasta in a large pot of boiling water until just tender. Before draining, reserve ½ cup of the water. Drain the pasta and place in a large bowl. Add the tomato mixture, reserved split peas and enough of the pasta water to moisten. Sprinkle with the Parmesan.

Serves 4

Per serving: 395 calories, 9.3 grams fat (21% of calories), 4.2 grams dietary fiber, 16 grams protein, 63.6 grams carbohydrate, 2 milligrams cholesterol, 392 milligrams sodium. Also a very good source of niacin, thiamine, folate and vitamin C.

Split-Pea and Spinach Soup with Garlic Yogurt

2 cups chopped onions
1 cup diced carrots
1 tablespoon chopped garlic
2 tablespoons olive oil
2 cups green split peas, sorted and rinsed
9 cups water or defatted chicken stock (or a mixture)
1 box (10 ounces) frozen chopped spinach, thawed but not drained
1 tablespoon lemon juice
    Dash of hot-pepper sauce
1 cup low-fat yogurt
1 large clove garlic, minced

In a Dutch oven or 4-quart saucepan, combine the onions, carrots, chopped garlic and 1 tablespoon of the oil. Cook, stirring occasionally, over medium-low heat until the vegetables begin to sizzle. Reduce the heat to low and cook, stirring often, for 15 minutes, or until the onions turn golden.

Add the split peas and water or stock. Increase the heat to medium-high and bring to a boil. Reduce the heat to medium-low, cover the pan and cook for 1 hour.

Stir in the spinach. Cook, uncovered, for 30 minutes, or until the split peas are tender and the soup is very thick. Remove from the heat and allow to cool for about 5 minutes. Stir in the lemon juice and hot-pepper sauce.

Transfer about ⅓ of the soup to a blender and process until smooth. Pour back into the pan.

In a small bowl, whisk together the yogurt, minced garlic and the remaining 1 tablespoon oil.

Serve the soup topped with dollops of the garlic yogurt.

Serves 8

Per serving: 245 calories, 4.5 grams fat (17% of calories), 5.1 grams dietary fiber, 15.1 grams protein, 38.2 grams carbohydrate, 2 milligrams cholesterol, 103 milligrams sodium. Also a very good source of folate and vitamin A.

Beautiful You

24   Spots Away

How to remove skin spots and stop them from returning.

Age spots. Liver spots. It doesn't matter what you call them—they add unnecessary years to your complexion. They're the reason that your hands give away your age. But nowadays you can do more about spots than simply count them as they appear. Here's how.

Identify the Problem

Freckles, age spots and melasma (dark patches that can appear with pregnancy) are all common types of hyperpigmentation (flat brownish blotches caused when your skin produces too much melanin). Hyperpigmentation can have different causes, but one element that plays a part in all is your skin's overexposure to the sun.

When you repeatedly expose unprotected skin to the sun, it tries to protect itself by producing an overabundance of melanin (the pigmented cells in your skin) in uneven patches.

Age spots are the most common type of hyperpigmentation and are more properly called solar lentigos. These frecklelike spots have nothing to do with the functioning of your liver and little to do with age. Although they commonly appear in adulthood, their primary cause is accumulated sun damage.

How to tell whether you have freckles or solar lentigos? "Freckles appear when you're young, they're worse in the summer and they tend to fade with age," says Nicholas J. Lowe, M.D., clinical professor of dermatology at the University of California, Los Angeles, School of Medicine. "Solar lentigos are generally larger, less regular in shape and darker than freckles, and appear only on areas that suffered from sun exposure, like the backs of your hands or your face."

"While both freckles and solar lentigos are harmless, they can be confused with more serious brown spots that are precancerous lesions," says John E. Wolf Jr., M.D., professor and chairman of the Dermatology Department at Baylor College of Medicine in Houston. "If a brown spot pops up out of the blue, or an old one suddenly changes shape, becomes raised or bleeds, have a dermatologist look at it to be certain it's not an early melanoma," the potentially fatal form of skin cancer that is increasing more rapidly than any other type of cancer.

A dermatologist can evaluate the various types of hyperpigmentation to identify your age spots correctly and be certain that they're benign, says Dr. Lowe. "The earlier a melanoma is found and treated, the better the chance of a complete cure."

Another type of benign hyperpigmentation that can resemble solar lentigos are the pigmented blotches called melasma, which frequently appear during pregnancy or when a woman is on birth control pills. (Men can have them, too, but it's much more unusual.)

A melasma, like a freckle or age spot, is a benign flat discoloration but covers a larger area, most commonly on the face. The color can vary from light to dark brown, depending on your original skin color. The condition can go away on its own, although its disappearance may be very gradual. Even if you decide not to treat melasma, Dr. Wolf suggests always wearing a sunscreen.

First-Line Antispot Tactics

Your very first step toward clearer skin is prevention of further damage. "The only way to stop blotches in their tracks is by sensible sun protection," says Dr. Lowe.

"Start using an SPF 15 (or higher) sunscreen on a daily basis," says Dr. Wolf. "Apply it to the backs of your hands and to your face first thing in the morning before you put on any moisturizer or makeup. When you wash your hands, don't forget to reapply your sunscreen. If you see the beginnings of age spots or melasma, switch to a higher SPF sunscreen than the one you're currently using."

"You must be willing to take preventive measures against future sun damage," says Dr. Lowe. "If you're not prepared to use a sunscreen that has an SPF of 15 or higher and that blocks both UVA and UVB rays, there's really no point in my removing your spots, because in a number of months your skin will be back in the same shape it was when you first came to see me. Prevention must begin the moment you walk out of my office."

Light discolorations, especially on the face, can sometimes be concealed with makeup. But there are also ways to fade them. "Your most sensible first step is over-the-counter skin-bleaching agents that contain hydroquinone," says Dr. Wolf. Hydroquinone works by interfering with your skin's production of the precursors of melanin, so the spots don't reform as your skin sloughs off old layers.

The level of hydroquinone in OTC products, however, is low compared with the concentration a dermatologist can prescribe and can take literally several months or even years to show a noticeable improvement.

"If you try one of the OTC bleaches," says Dr. Wolf, "I recommend you give it a chance for at least a few months. If you see absolutely no difference after using both a bleach and a sunscreen regularly, then you need to go to something stronger." And you have several options.

Your dermatologist can prescribe a higher concentration of hydroquinone either alone or in combination with Retin-A treatments. "For patients with very light solar lentigos, I may recommend a daily program that begins with a good sunscreen—that means one that blocks both UVA and UVB rays—applied half an hour before you go outside in the morning. Next use the hydroquinone," says Dr. Lowe. "This would be followed by Retin-A nightly or every other night, depending on their tolerance of it."

"Melasma is also treated with hydroquinone and/or Retin-A," adds Dr. Wolf. "Particularly in treating melasma, I may add a cortisone cream to that mixture to enhance the bleaching effect. The full-court press for melasma is Retin-A, hydroquinone and cortisone cream."

While this regimen is the most acceptable treatment for melasma, darker spots as well as those on your chest and hands probably will not respond as well to it. Also, this process is relatively slow to work. Even with this entire regimen working for you, it can take a year or more to see a cosmetically acceptable result.

There are two ways to treat solar lentigos using chemicals. One is to use trichloracetic acid (TCA), frequently used in chemical peels, to treat just the individual brown spots. "This might be the treatment of choice for someone who has just two or three little spots that aren't too dark," says Dr. Wolf. "These spots could also be frozen with liquid nitrogen."

One possible drawback to these methods is that it can be difficult to control the amount of lightening that takes place—leaving the dark spots too white. "Although acid peels and freezing are faster, they can result in hypopigmenting," says Dr. Wolf.

The Laser Option

"The best methods for actually removing age spots are the ruby laser and the flash lamp pumped dye pigmented laser, which are approved for such use by the Food and Drug Administration," says Dr. Lowe. "These lasers can be set to destroy only the pigment cells. The great thing about laser treatment for this problem is that in the hands of an expert, you don't run the risk of having white spots where the dark spots had been. Other methods such as electric surgery, cryotherapy or chemical peels run a greater risk of removing too much pigment. The only caveat is that, as with any surgery, it's only as good as the practitioner." Check to make sure the physician is trained in lasers and belongs to the American Society for Laser Medicine and Surgery.

"The lasers that are effective are those whose wavelengths of light are absorbed by the melanin," says Dr. Wolf. The major drawback of lasers is that they're the most expensive method of treatment. They also may have some of the same drawbacks as TCA peels or cryosurgery, but to a lesser degree.

After you've chosen your dermatologist for laser therapy, and you're both certain that all the dark spots you want removed are benign, what next?

"I give my patients information on the procedure and what to expect," says Dr. Lowe. "Next I test the laser at three different intensity levels on test sites that are typical of the growths or pigmented spots we want to remove. I explain that the pain is usually like the snap of a rubber band against your skin. Then we meet again in four weeks."

The laser procedure itself can usually be accomplished in one or two visits, depending on the individual skin, the number of spots treated and the darkness of the pigmentation. To treat one age spot the size of an eraser head usually takes a few seconds; it then clears over two to four weeks.

25 Ancient Traditions for Today's Woman

Tap the beautifying potential of Mother Nature's bounty.

These days, a trip to the beauty section of the local drugstore may leave you wondering whether you've accidentally sashayed into the gardening department. Shelves are abloom with botanical beautifiers that all promise great results stemming from their natural rather than synthetic ingredients.

While botanicals don't have the scientific research behind them that a product like Retin-A has, they have been the basic ingredient for skin-care favorites for centuries. This doesn't mean that they all work as tradition suggests (tradition has been known to be wrong about the effects of herbs and other natural substances), but many botanicals do seem to have some obvious cosmetic benefits. So for the novice to natural products, the question is: With the plethora of plant- and flower-based products, which botanical ingredients should you look for—and why?

Here's what a number of herbal experts came up with when they were asked to create a list of botanical all-stars—the herbal and floral ingredients they believe to be most effective for cosmetic purposes.

Botanical Basics

"Before I can advise which botanicals are best," says Pratima Raichur, an aesthetician (a cosmetologist specializing in skin) and founder of the Tej Salon in Manhattan, "it's essential to know about the various forms of each natural ingredient and how they are best used. An herbal extract is made from fresh herbs that are suspended in alcohol, then strained. This means the formula will be a bit drying and can be used on oily skin. Essential oils, which are derived from steaming and distilling herbs and flowers, are used to nourish the skin because their molecular density allows the oils to penetrate. Herbs that are found in powder form (which means they have been dried and crushed) are best when used to cleanse the skin."

When asked to choose a few of the most effective herbal ingredients, Raichur begins with sandalwood powder, noting its soothing effects. She recommends aloe vera for the same reason. Aloe can be found both in products and in its crushed-powder form at most health-food stores. Working as a purifier, it is an especially helpful ingredient to look for in acne masks.

Another favorite cited by Raichur is coriander, a spice derived from the seeds of cilantro and found in most supermarkets. "Coriander," says Raichur, "is very effective for both cooling and soothing."

Oils derived from nuts are also highly favored by Raichur for their skin-nourishing properties. For a homemade mask for dry skin, Raichur suggests grinding almonds or sunflower seeds and adding a few drops of milk until the mixture becomes pasty. Be sure the nuts have been ground to a superfine powder with no slivers that might scratch. She then says to apply the hydrating mixture (don't rub it in) and leave it on for half an hour.

Raichur mentions a number of essential oils she

219

finds highly effective. "Sandalwood, jasmine and rose have calming properties and should be used on dry, sensitive skin, while lavender and sage oils are best for oily skin. These essential oils can be found in skin-care products and, in their pure form, at health-food stores."

Several botanic-based aestheticians believe that rosemary is very refreshing to use as an all-over herbal wash. They use it as a hair rinse to counteract the residue left by synthetic materials used on the hair. Lavender, on the other hand, is regarded as especially soothing. Other botanical ingredients favored by those who use botanicals include: citrus extracts, which will degrease the skin; rose, which has hydrating properties; and chamomile, which acts as an anti-inflammatory.

Raichur notes that people looking for natural products should be sure to read all labels. "If the ingredients contain a long list of chemicals and just a few herbal extracts, this product is not natural."

Just as not all products that are advertised as natural really qualify, it's also important to remember that if you have a rash or other physical skin eruption, your first line of attack should be to consult a physician.

Natural ingredients aren't always better than synthetic ones. In fact, they're sometimes more likely to cause allergic skin reactions. Lime, for example, can cause "photosensitivity." That means that, when exposed to lime and sunlight simultaneously, skin absorbs more radiant energy than normal. The result is a blotchy, sunburned effect. So, while botanicals can offer delightful cosmetic benefits, for true therapeutic needs, check with your dermatologist.

Herbs for Your Hair

"Healthy and beautiful hair through plants" is the philosophy on which the French company Phyto-thérathrie was created. Its founder and owner is Patrick Ales, whose passion for hair and botany led him to formulate a line of botanically based hair-care products now available in the United States.

Says company spokeswoman Anna Lempereur,

"Over 100 plants, flower extracts and oils are used in our products. Some of those that we have found to be the most effective include jojoba, which rehydrates dry hair and nourishes its keratin content; rosemary, which acts as a toner and regulates the scalp's sebaceous (oil-producing) glands; calendula, a flower that moisturizes hair as well as soothes and calms the scalp; and garlic and horseradish extracts, which act as natural, non-chemical relaxers that coat and smooth hair, making it more manageable."

Lempereur also cites the beneficial properties of beetroot extract: "Because of its high sugar content, when beet root is distilled, it ferments into a natural alcohol, which, when used in styling sprays, we find is less drying than synthetic alcohol."

Botanicals Go Mainstream

The Body Shop, which has stores in over 40 countries around the world, is another company founded on the use of naturally based products. A wide range of floral and herbal essences and extracts are found in the entire range of their products. Some of founder Anita Roddick's favorites include aloe-vera gel, which Roddick likes for its healing and anti-inflammatory properties; elderflower, which acts as a natural astringent and is supposed to reduce under-eye puffiness; chamomile; peppermint oil, which contains menthol and has both astringent and antiseptic properties; and rose, which, if distilled in water or used in its oil form, has relaxing and cleansing properties.

Joe Gubernick, senior vice president of research and development for Estée Lauder Companies, is hard-pressed to mention any favorite herbs used in their Origins product line because "each of the more than 75 herbs we use has a special function, and when used in conjunction with other herbs, brings balance to the skin and body."

However, he is willing to cite some of the ingredients used most often and why. "Egyptian geranium," says Gubernick, "is strongly stimulating to the skin; French clary sage is rich in plant hormones and has an ener-

221

gizing effect on the skin." Gubernick also mentions lavender and rosemary for their soothing effect.

While ancient folklore provides insight into time-honored traditions, even modern-day women who trust cosmetic chemists more than chamomile creams use and enjoy many of these botanicals for their wonderful fragrance alone.

26   Enriching "Pore" Skin

Simple tips to make your skin shine.

Do you wish your pores were smaller? Many people do—and rue the fact that they can't shrink the size of the pores they were born with. The good news is that even though you can't change nature's design specifications, doctors and skin-care specialists agree you can take steps to make pores appear smaller.

Here's what you need to know to ensure that your pores are healthy and barely apparent.

Pore Basics

Beneath the surface of the skin are sebaceous (oil-producing) glands. The openings of these glands, which are located on the skin's surface, are your pores. A pore becomes more noticeable when it stretches to secrete higher volumes of oil that are produced beneath the skin's surface.

Enlarged pores are most commonly found on the lower forehead, nose and chin area. According to Amy Newburger, M.D., a dermatologist and assistant professor at Columbia Presbyterian Hospital in New York City, "These facial areas are prone to enlarged pores because directly underneath them are the largest oil glands associated with the face. Because these glands produce a higher volume of oil, a larger pore is required to drain all of the oil being secreted."

A pore's visibility is increased if the oil doesn't drain properly or if surface oil is allowed to accumulate. Part of the reason is that body oil is oxidized and then becomes discolored. Excess oil also means blackheads and an oily sheen on the surface of the skin.

What to Do

So the key is keeping your skin free of debris and minimizing the amount of oil on your skin. Here are some tips from dermatologists and skin-care experts on how to do just that.

Cleanse ▶ Experts agree that your first plan of attack should be a diligent but careful approach to cleansing. John F. Romano, M.D., clinical assistant professor of medicine in dermatology at the New York Hospital–Cornell Medical Center in New York City, suggests cleansing one to three times a day with a mild soap. If your skin is sensitive, cleanse only at night and just rinse with lukewarm water in the morning.

He advises against using cleansing brushes, cleaning grains and abrasive sponges, all of which may generate further irritation. Rather, he suggests cleansing with a soft, freshly laundered washcloth.

Alan Shalita, M.D., chairman of the Dermatology Department at the State University of New York Health Science Center at Brooklyn, also suggests gentle cleansing as a remedy for acne-prone skin. "However," he says, "if at-home cleansing does not produce satisfactory results, it may be due to pores that are plugged up." In this case, Dr. Shalita suggests going to a reputable aesthetician (a cosmetologist specializing in skin) or a dermatologist or dermatologist's assistant for a deep-cleaning treatment.

"One thing you shouldn't do," says Dr. Newburger, "is squeeze the affected areas. This should not be done under any circumstances. Squeezing these sensitive areas can lead to permanent scarring if areas become inflamed or infected. It can cause the blood vessel network in these areas to appear more prominent and can even cause permanently enlarged pores."

Use Astringents and Toners ▶ Some dermatologists and aestheticians agree that toners and astringents can help to lessen the exaggerated appearance of enlarged pores by removing debris that collects on skin and by minimizing facial oil.

Pratima Raichur, aesthetician and founder of the Tej Salon in Manhattan, says, "Before you rush out to purchase an astringent or toner, check your medicine chest and refrigerator. I find that witch hazel, yogurt and buttermilk are all very effective when used to cleanse and remove oil from the skin."

If none of these treatments appeals to you, Raichur suggests concocting your own solution from citrus juice and water. Says Raichur, "Two ounces of water combined with one teaspoon of lemon juice can be used to make a mild and refreshing facial astringent."

If you prefer the laboratory-formulated, store-bought variety of skin treatments, Dr. Newburger suggests you look for a toner or astringent that contains the ingredient salicylic acid. "Salicylic acid will dissolve dead skin and skin flakes without increasing sensitivity to the sun," she says. "It also gives the skin a polished look."

Try Facial Masks ▶ Many cosmetic companies offer masks formulated specifically to reduce the appearance of enlarged pores. Be aware, however, that no permanent solution exists in a tube or in a bottle. These masks work on reducing the appearance of enlarged pores, not on shrinking the size of the pores themselves.

Like traditional cleansers and astringents, masks will help to unclog debris-plugged pores and absorb excess oil found on the surface of the skin. As for the benefits of a mask versus those of an astringent or toner, Alex Znaiden, who is director of skin-care research and development at Avon, says, "An astringent helps to remove surface oils and dirt, but a pore mask is designed to clean down inside the pores."

When choosing a mask, avoid the peel-off variety.

Dr. Newburger says this type of mask is relaxing and can make skin seem smoother, but it is not as oil-absorbent and therefore not as effective in minimizing the appearance of enlarged pores.

Moisturize ▶ More well informed than ever about what it takes to care for healthy skin, women today are already aware of the benefits to be had from using a moisturizer as part of a daily skin-care regimen. It's important, however, to choose your moisturizer in accordance with your skin type. Many women will wrongly assume they have oily skin because enlarged pores are a problem on one area of the face. In fact, you can have enlarged pores and have combination skin or even dry skin.

When selecting a moisturizer, look for one that specifies a formulation for your skin type on the label. If you want a moisturizer that doubles as a treatment for enlarged pores, Dr. Romano suggests choosing one that will also act as a mild exfoliant. "Look for a moisturizer that contains a lactic acid. This ingredient will act as a mild peel on the uppermost layer of skin and make enlarged pores appear less prominent," says Dr. Romano.

Keep Diet in Perspective ▶ Contrary to popular belief, you can't directly modify your skin through diet. Says Dr. Romano, "Body oil is manufactured inside the skin. It is not absorbed from what you eat." This is not to say that diet doesn't matter. All experts strongly suggest maintaining a balanced diet for optimum internal and external health.

Fight the Age Factor ▶ Surprisingly, it's not uncommon for people to develop enlarged pores after age 50. "Once past the age of 50, the skin's oil production can be irregular," says Dr. Newburger. "And one isolated sebaceous gland can become enlarged even as oil production elsewhere is decreased." This can result in localized areas of sebaceous hyperplasia (when the general area around the oil gland becomes raised). To combat the problem, Dr. Newburger recommends being

225

extremely gentle when cleansing your face. She also advises using a facial mask, but not more than two or three times a week.

Consider Professional Treatment ▶ If you've tried all the suggestions listed above and remain unhappy with the results, it may be time to consult a dermatologist, who can prescribe a more intensive treatment.

Your doctor's recommendations might include the use of Retin-A, a mild chemical peel or an alpha hydroxy acid (made from fruit and vegetable pulp), which is found in doctor-prescribed creams.

All these treatments will cause a mild peeling on the skin's surface, remove debris and make enlarged pores seem less noticeable.

Conceal ▶ In addition to whatever treatment you choose, cosmetics can also help conceal enlarged pores. Mickey Mikawa, a professional makeup artist at the Vartali Salon in Manhattan, says that because enlarged pores often result in an oily sheen, your makeup routine should be similar to one used by women who have oily skin, although you should choose products suited to your skin type.

Before applying makeup, Mikawa suggests using an astringent to remove any additional oil found on the skin's surface. "Next," says Mikawa, "apply an oil-free moisturizer formulated for your type of skin. Then, using a sponge to keep makeup application even, apply a light, liquid, oil-free foundation.

"This will create a smooth canvas for makeup and absorb excess oil to keep skin from shining. After this, dust the face with loose powder to hold makeup in place."

When applying color to the cheek area, Mikawa recommends using a powder rather than a cream blush. "A powder will not be absorbed into skin as readily as a cream that contains oil," says Mikawa. "When it comes to touch-ups, first blot the entire face with a tissue, then reapply compact or loose powder. And don't forget to gently and thoroughly cleanse your skin every night to remove the day's buildup of makeup and oils."

Mind
and
Body

27 Conquering Depression

It isn't all in your mind.

In late November, Pennsylvania accountant David Ferguson started feeling blue.

Really blue.

He'd drag himself around, feeling depressed and anxious. He'd have trouble sleeping. And he'd start overeating on a major scale. His depression continued for months. And the thing was, he had no idea why—there was nothing in his life to be so deeply depressed about.

What was wrong with his mind? he wondered. Why was he so depressed?

Finally, in desperation, David contacted a local psychiatrist who listened to his symptoms, did some tests and realized that his depression was caused by a physical disorder—actually the body's response to a sunlight deficiency—that afflicts 5 to 25 million people a year. David was treated and soon had more energy than he'd had in months. And over the next several weeks he even started losing his extra weight. What a relief!

And that's the good news about depression: Nearly one-third of all people diagnosed with it may actually be suffering from a physical illness masquerading as an emotional problem. Solve the physical problem, and in most cases the depression goes away.

This is so even though ongoing, unexplained (so-called chronic) depression is a major health problem and can seem (to the sufferer) hopeless. It can disrupt a person's normal routine, causing lack of sleep and bringing on feelings of fatigue, inability to concentrate, changes in appetite and more.

There are as many as 75 hidden physical causes of chronic depression, says Mark Gold, M.D., author of *The Good News about Depression* and a pioneer in the field of physically caused depression. Dr. Gold says the best way to uncover these causes is a comprehensive physical examination, including a complete patient history and a battery of standard medical tests. And he urges depressed people or their families and friends to locate "biopsychiatrists" who understand the "medical mimickers" of major depression.

Here are ten of the most commonly identified physical reasons behind these mental consequences.

Prescription Problems

The very same drugs that boost your health may also cause depression. But correcting the problem may be as simple as changing drugs or adjusting your dosage.

Doctors are now generally aware that drugs may indeed have depressive side effects, says Arthur I. Jacknowitz, Pharm.D., professor of clinical pharmacy at the West Virginia University School of Pharmacy in Morgantown. In fact, it may be the first thing they consider with patients on regular medications who come to them complaining of depression.

So don't try to tough it out. Seek help right away, says Stuart C. Yudofsky, M.D., chairman of the Department of Psychiatry and behavioral sciences of Baylor College of Medicine in Houston. "If you're depressed, no matter what the cause, you and your doctor should take it very seriously."

Symptoms of depression may not surface right away, says Dr. Jacknowitz. If you've been taking a medication for six months to a year and then begin to experience the blues, it could still be your medication. On the other hand, don't automatically assume that a drug is causing your depression just because it's on a list of drugs with that possible side effect. Depression usually occurs in only a small percentage of the people taking any given drug.

Here, in a nutshell, are descriptions of the major categories of prescription drugs known to cause depression in some people.

Antihypertensives ▶ If you have high blood pressure, you may be taking reserpine, methyldopa, clonidine or beta-blockers. All of these may cause some symptoms of

229
∎

depression. Dr. Yudofsky, author of *What You Need to Know about Psychiatric Drugs*, says most patients know when it's the drug that's causing the depression, but other factors may be compounding the problem.

Dr. Yudofsky considers a group of antihypertensives known as ACE inhibitors to be free of depressive side effects. These include Capoten, Vasotec, Zestril and Prinivil.

Heart Medications ▶ Antiarrhythmic drugs are used to stabilize an erratic heartbeat and to treat congestive heart failure. Digitalis, one of the most commonly prescribed antiarrhythmics, does cause depression in some people. Other antiarrhythmics may not have this same effect, and your doctor may decide to switch medications.

Cortisone and Similar Steroids ▶ If you have asthma, arthritis, psoriasis, severe allergies, colitis or one of a number of other ailments, you may be taking cortisone or other corticosteroids orally. These drugs are known to cause depression in some people.

If you suspect that corticosteroids may be causing your symptoms of depression, talk to your doctor about the options. Other nonsteroidal drugs may be available. In some cases, corticosteroids applied to the skin may be effective without depressive side effects. But do not discontinue your medication without your doctor's supervision. Stopping corticosteroids suddenly can lead to a very serious condition called Addison's disease.

Glaucoma Medication ▶ Timolol, one of the beta-blockers used to treat high blood pressure, is also used in eyedrop form to treat glaucoma. And in both cases, the drug may lead to symptoms of depression.

Antihistamines ▶ Antihistamines are commonly prescribed for allergic symptoms, including runny nose, itchy eyes, sneezing and itchy skin. If you have hay fever or other allergies, you may be taking antihistamines for months at a time. "After long-term antihistamine therapy, you're just out of sorts. You feel tired. You feel fatigued. And that could lead to depression," says Dr. Jacknowitz. In that case, you may want to discuss the newer, nonsedating antihistamines with your doctor.

Thyroid Trouble

More than seven million Americans suffer from thyroid problems. And thyroid malfunctions are a major cause of depression. In fact, says Dr. Gold, 10 to 15 percent of all depressed patients have some form of thyroid disease.

Fortunately, there are simple blood tests for detecting problems in thyroid function, including the T4 test and the thyroid-stimulating hormone test (TSH). The tests can determine whether you suffer from hypothyroidism, the most common thyroid disorder to be linked with depression, as well as other thyroid dysfunctions.

In hypothyroidism, your thyroid gland secretes too little hormone, and your metabolism slows. You may then experience a range of symptoms, including weight gain, dry skin, hair loss and constipation. Also, your sleep patterns will change. You may find yourself fatigued and sleeping more than usual. Your interest in sex may plummet. Yet many people with an underactive thyroid don't even know it. The Thyroid Foundation of America estimates that half of all people with hypothyroidism are undiagnosed or misdiagnosed.

Many hypothyroid patients are significantly depressed during the course of the disease. After the problem is diagnosed, treatment is available. The most common treatment is a synthetic thyroid hormone, taken orally.

The Monthly Blues

Most women suffer from some form of premenstrual syndrome (PMS), but about 5 percent experience depression so severe that it disrupts their daily lives. Symptoms include mood swings, food cravings, crying and insomnia.

It shouldn't be surprising: A woman's body is buffeted by a hormonal whirlwind just prior to menstruation. Progesterone and estrogen levels rise and fall, and endorphins (as well as other hormones associated with mood) change during this time.

Researchers theorize that when a woman's estrogen levels rise during the menstrual cycle, the level of vitamin B_6, or pyridoxine, may change. Since B_6 is involved in the body's production of mood-lifting neurotransmitters like serotonin, low levels of it may cause mild depression.

Dietary sources of vitamin B_6 include chicken, fish, rice and whole-wheat products. Supplemental B_6 may help, says Barbara Parry, M.D., associate professor of psychiatry at the University of California at San Diego. Be careful not to exceed ten milligrams per day, however. Excess vitamin B_6 can cause nerve damage.

Judith Wurtman, Ph.D., a nutritional researcher at the Massachusetts Institute of Technology, believes that a diet high in complex carbohydrates, such as pasta and potatoes, may also beat PMS-related depression by boosting serotonin levels. And other doctors say that many of their patients with PMS have reported improvements in their condition after eating a diet that's high in carbohydrates.

Other Hormonal Shifts

PMS may be the most frequent reminder that a woman's reproductive hormones are often out of balance. But there are three other common hormonal disturbances that can lead to depression in women.

Menopause ▶ "Several articles have been written about the 'myth of depression at menopause.' I think *that's* a myth," says Dr. Parry. The "menopause blues" really do exist for some women. Fortunately, the problem is very treatable, she adds.

Symptoms of this type of depression usually reach a peak at around the age of 50 or 51, at the onset of menopause, when most women have their very last period. And the depression is not just an emotional reaction to the loss of their ability to bear children.

A woman's estrogen level drops at menopause, and some researchers theorize that this lack of estrogen might cause changes in other hormones or chemicals in the brain such as serotonin, which has been linked to mood disorders.

Evidence suggests that regular, vigorous exercise can counteract the effects of this drop in serotonin by generally raising the level of good-humor hormones circulating in your blood.

Estrogen replacement therapy alone may not relieve the symptoms of menopausal depression. However, if your symptoms are severe, it may be a necessary first step to further treatment. That's because antidepressant drugs won't work in the face of low estrogen levels. Estrogen replacement therapy raises estrogen levels, making it possible to use antidepressants.

For mild depression, no treatment may be necessary. But ask your doctor to evaluate your situation and recommend treatment options.

Oral Contraceptives ▶ The Pill is the most popular reversible contraceptive method in America. Yet up to 50 percent of the women who stop using oral contraceptives do it because of feelings of depression caused by the contraceptive.

Most depressive side effects are related to the dosage of the hormones estrogen and progestin contained in the Pill. So talk to your family doctor or gynecologist about the depression you're experiencing and ask if you can be given a different dosage.

The high levels of estrogen in many contraceptive pills may also inhibit the levels of vitamin B_6 found in certain predisposed PMS sufferers, says Dr. Parry. Again, supplemental B_6 may be helpful in some women with mild symptoms, under a doctor's supervision.

Postpartum Depression ▶ Like PMS and depression induced by oral contraceptives, the so-called baby blues may also be triggered by changing levels of reproductive hormones. During pregnancy, depression is uncommon. But during the first month after the baby is born, the incidence of depression shoots up dramatically and stays up for six months. Fifty to 80 percent of all mothers experience the baby blues, which are characterized by crying, rapid mood shifts and irritability.

First-time mothers are especially at risk. So are women with a history of depression. There are treatment options your doctor can recommend, including antidepressant medications for those who are seriously depressed.

High Sugar Levels

Could you be one of the nearly seven million Americans who have diabetes but don't yet know it? If so, the depression you experience may be caused by this untreated condition. And even if you know that you have diabetes, depression may result if you don't control the disease by a special diet or insulin shots or pills.

Insulin is the body's sugar delivery van. When too little insulin is produced, or when the body can't use it properly, sugar pools in the blood instead of being delivered to cells where it's needed for energy. This high level of blood sugar can lead to low energy, fatigue and sleeplessness, which in turn can lead to depression. If your problem is, in fact, diabetes, these depressive symptoms may be accompanied by increased urination and excessive hunger and thirst.

To diagnose your condition, your doctor may measure your glucose (blood sugar) levels or perform a glucose tolerance test. (After an overnight fast, a sugary, high-glucose beverage is given, then blood is drawn at regular intervals to track blood sugar levels.)

Just the opposite of diabetes, hypoglycemia (which is caused by too little sugar in the blood) causes symptoms ranging from weakness and nervousness to shallow breathing, confusion and rapid heartbeat. Some diabetes patients experience hypoglycemia when they overdose on insulin or skip a meal, which shunts too much sugar out of the blood.

Rapid-Weight-Loss Diets

If you're on a diet that leaves you hungry, you're bound to get depressed, says George L. Blackburn, M.D., Ph.D., chief of the Nutrition/Metabolism Laboratory with the Cancer Research Institute at New England Deaconess Hospital in Boston and associate professor at Harvard Medical School.

"For every person who's depressed, there'd be a lot more if there were no food! Food is one of the great tranquilizers. Food is mostly the solution," he says. And when you're on a crash diet and getting too little food, you're on the road to what Dr. Blackburn calls "brain pain," a complex mix of factors that boils down to the fact that your mind and body are in pain from lack of food.

So depression may be a warning sign that you're pushing your diet too far, too fast. Not only will that leave you feeling depressed, the depression itself is likely to sabotage your diet as well, says Dr. Blackburn.

That's why he recommends an adequate, healthy diet that satisfies you and doesn't leave you feeling hungry. "If the diet you're on makes you feel hungry, it's not going to work. So stop doing it and establish a healthy diet with a lot of fluid and fiber, and it's going to be grazing—eating five to six times a day."

Lack of Exercise

Research has shown that a lack of exercise can be an independent risk factor for moderate depression, especially among women. Regardless of other factors like household income or employment status, those with low activity levels were at significantly greater risk for depression.

Researchers at the Human Population Laboratory of the California Department of Health Services surveyed 6,928 residents of Alameda County, California, and found that the link between lack of exercise and depression also exists for men. And their findings suggest something very positive: When inactive people finally do start exercising, they are less likely to have depressive symptoms.

"Just as quitting smoking can lower your risk of lung

235

disease, it appears that beginning to exercise can actually reduce your risk of depression—even if you were a couch potato," says Terry Camacho, research analyst and coauthor of the Alameda County study.

Dark Moods

The accountant described at the beginning of this story was suffering from a condition known as seasonal affective disorder, or SAD. SAD victims exhibit all the classic symptoms of chronic depression—all because of too little sunlight in the fall and winter.

Millions of Americans suffer from SAD, says Dan Oren, M.D., a senior clinical investigator in the Clinical Psychobiology Branch of the National Institute of Mental Health. And 83 percent of those afflicted with SAD are women between the ages of 30 and 50. So don't rule it out, even if you haven't noticed a cycle to your depression—especially since it can be treated quite effectively.

Doctors feel that some people with SAD may have an ultrasensitivity to a hormone called melatonin. In darker months, melatonin levels are high because this hormone is only produced at night or in the absence of light. In the presence of light, melatonin secretion is inhibited.

So the first-line treatment for SAD is light therapy administered by specially trained health professionals. During light therapy, you are exposed to regular sessions of bright, full-spectrum light that are basically equivalent to looking out of a window on a clear spring day with lots of sun. The sessions usually range from half an hour to six hours daily, depending on the intensity of the light and the severity of the depression.

Nutritional Shortfalls

"Anytime the body doesn't get enough of a nutrient, activity levels are impaired, which can mimic depression and be labeled as such," says David Levitsky, Ph.D., professor of nutrition and psychology at Cornell University in Ithaca, New York.

However, there has been little research into the

emotional effects of mild nutritional deficiencies. And severe deficiencies—leading to major depression—are rare. Still, preliminary research indicates that a number of vitamin and mineral deficiencies may lead to symptoms of depression. Several likely possibilities are discussed below. If you suspect a deficiency, talk to your doctor.

Iron ▶ Advanced cases of iron-deficiency anemia can lead to feeling depressed, listless and lethargic, says Ernesto Pollitt, Ph.D., professor of human development at the University of California at Davis. Countless clinical reports by doctors suggest that even mild anemia may have a similar effect on mood. Unfortunately, says Dr. Pollitt, there is simply no research that's been done to document this. But, he says, "if you are tired, listless and apathetic in a way you're not used to, you'd better check your iron levels"—especially if you have medical problems that could affect iron levels. The problem can be diagnosed with a hemoglobin test.

Thiamine ▶ In older people, even marginal deficiencies of thiamine can lead to weight loss, sleep disturbances, inactivity, irritability and depression. In a study of 80 older Irish women with moderate thiamine deficiency, thiamine supplements improved their sleep patterns, decreased fatigue and restored appetite and general well-being. The authors of the study, from the Department of Nutrition at the University of California at Davis, recommend having your thiamine levels checked (with a blood test) if you are over 65 and experiencing these symptoms of depression. The Recommended Dietary Allowance (RDA) for thiamine is 1.5 milligrams for men and 1.1 milligrams for women.

Selenium ▶ Even moderately low levels of selenium may result in a low mood, anxiety and tiredness. Researchers at the University College, Swansea, Wales, found that when dietary intake of selenium went down, reports of anxiety, depression and tiredness went up. The good news: Supplements of 100 micrograms of selenium per day improved mood and anxiety levels. The

237

RDA for selenium in men is 70 micrograms, and for women it's 55 micrograms.

Magnesium ▶ Low magnesium is very common, says Daniel Kanofsky, M.D., assistant professor of psychiatry at the Albert Einstein College of Medicine in New York City. Its symptoms can include depression, irritability and confusion. There is not yet enough evidence, however, to conclude that supplementing with magnesium can alleviate these symptoms. If you suspect a magnesium deficiency, get a blood test to confirm it.

In some fascinating but preliminary studies, low magnesium levels were also found to be present in sufferers of chronic fatigue syndrome. In one of those studies, injections of magnesium sulfate significantly improved energy level and emotional status. More research is definitely needed to confirm these findings.

Questionable Food Combinations

If you always eat your complex carbohydrates—like rice, bread and cereal—together with some protein source, you may be at risk for mild depression, says Dr. Wurtman, author of *Managing Your Mind and Mood through Food*.

She speculates that that's because the amino acids in protein prevent tryptophan from getting into the brain. And tryptophan is essential for producing serotonin, the brain chemical that keeps your moods stable. Her theory is that when eaten alone, complex carbohydrates boost serotonin production in the brain.

"This theory certainly holds up in animal studies," says Harry Gwirtsman, M.D., chief of the Mood Disorders Program at the National Institute of Mental Health. "But it still has not been shown to be true in humans. We need further research to help clarify it."

Dr. Wurtman recommends getting at least one meal a day that is very high in complex carbohydrates, with little or no protein. Rice, potatoes and plain pasta are good choices, but fruits won't work. They contain simple sugars, which don't stimulate serotonin release and that ensuing calming effect.

Sshhh! 28

Reducing noise levels can turn down the volume on stress, blood pressure and headaches.

Like fingernails across a chalkboard, so are the noises of our—*skkrreeeettcchhhh!!!*—lives.

On a typical day, you're jolted from sleep by a blaring alarm clock, jostled in your car by a cacophony of grinding-screeching-honking road noises, then jarred by a sudden siren wail and the deafening jangle of a jackhammer. And it's not even 9 A.M.

At work, you're practically numb to the drone of office equipment, the pounding of heavy machinery or the clicking of computer keyboards. At home, your teenager's taste for rock and rap comes in loud and clear. Even on weekends, your home sanctuary is invaded by yapping dogs and the ubiquitous roar of leaf blowers. Is it any wonder you feel so rattled?

Audiologists don't think so. Years ago, they suggested that the impact of noise pollution may go far beyond hearing loss. Now mounting research would have us believe that's true. While the research is not yet strong enough to prove cause and effect, intrusive, discordant sounds have been linked to stress, high blood pressure, learning disorders and more.

"Noise is taken for granted," says Evelyn Talbott, Ph.D., associate professor of epidemiology at the University of Pittsburgh Graduate School of Public Health. "But virtually all the research on the physiological effects of noise has found a correlation between noise and health problems."

Noise may not have to be loud enough to hurt your hearing to have a rebound effect on other systems in your body, some experts say. Studies have found suspected noise-related health problems—particularly hypertension—even when there's no hint of noise-induced hearing loss. But the good news is, you don't have to be a victim of your environment. There are ways you can protect yourself from the sounds that not only hurt your ears but that also may be sabotaging your health.

Noise and Your Heart

Recent research on what noise can do to your health—and the biological processes by which it may cause health problems—is scarce. That's due, in part, to cutbacks in federal funding for noise-abatement programs in the early 1980s. And noise is so pervasive that its effects are difficult to study. It's hard to measure exposure levels and to find control groups—people who've been isolated from noise or exposed at lower levels—as a basis of comparison.

But despite those limitations, most experts say there's enough evidence to convince them that chronic exposure to loud noise can be harmful, especially to your heart.

"The consensus in the field is that excessive noise may increase your risk of hypertension and other cardio-vascular diseases by about 10 percent," says Shirley Thompson, Ph.D., associate professor of epidemiology at the University of South Carolina in Columbia. Compared with the impact of other risk factors, like smoking, excess weight, a family history of heart problems and lack of exercise, that's not much. But if you're already at risk for heart problems, a 10 percent increase could be something to be concerned about, Dr. Thompson says.

What first forced scientists to sit up and take notice were studies on monkeys exposed to typical workplace noise, conducted by Ernest Peterson, Ph.D., associate professor of otolaryngology (ear, nose and throat medicine) at the University of Miami.

In a small study conducted in 1981, rhesus monkeys heard sounds simulating a construction site—bulldozers, pile-driving equipment and the like—24 hours a day for a period of nine months. Blood pressure readings taken during the din were 16 to 42 percent higher than those recorded before the experiment began. The results also showed that the noise-exposed monkeys had higher heart rates and pressure in their arteries—another indication their hearts were working harder during the noisy phase of the study. What's more, their blood pressures were still elevated when researchers followed up 27 days after the noise ended.

None of the monkeys in Dr. Peterson's studies experienced significant hearing loss because of noise exposure. "The processes of hearing loss and nonauditory damage may be independent," Dr. Peterson says. "So earplugs might protect your hearing, but there's no guarantee they'll protect you from these nonauditory effects."

There's also no guarantee that noise affects humans the same way it affects monkeys, Dr. Peterson says. But most of the studies done with humans also suggest that chronic exposure to loud noise in the workplace may raise blood pressure and cause other changes in the way your heart works. One, a study of 316 shipyard workers, showed that people working in a noisy environment had twice the risk of high blood pressure as those in a not-so-noisy environment. And that difference remained after classic risk factors for high blood pressure like age and body-fat-to-muscle ratio were taken into account.

But whether noise-induced blood pressure jumps occur in the absence of hearing loss is still a matter of debate. In fact, a study conducted by Dr. Talbott at the University of Pittsburgh measured the blood pressures and hearing abilities of 240 retired factory workers who had an average of 30 years of on-the-job noise exposure. There was no significant relationship between hearing loss and high blood pressure among the younger workers, aged 56 to 63. But more than half of the men aged 64 to 68 who had severe, noise-related hearing loss also had high blood pressure, and they were more likely to be on hypertension medication. Only 30 percent of the older men who didn't suffer hearing loss had high blood pressure.

A second study by Dr. Talbott's group yielded similar results.

"It's possible that there's a subset of people who are more susceptible to noise-induced hearing loss and noise-induced hypertension," she says.

It's obvious—and the experts agree—that more research is needed to clear up these issues. Says Dr. Thompson, "We need some long-term studies that follow

241

a population over time, in which only part of them are exposed to high noise levels, to see what proportion in each group develops elevated blood pressure."

Wired for Sound

Noise may also take a mental toll on you. Some studies suggest that children whose schools are in noisy areas score lower on tests than children in quieter schools. Irritability, aggressiveness, fatigue and lack of concentration have also been attributed to noise.

In one study, a researcher feigned a broken arm and dropped an armful of books. Nearby, another researcher was mowing a lawn. No passersby stopped to help the researcher as she struggled to retrieve her books. But when the experiment was repeated without the background noise of the lawn mower, several Good Samaritans stopped to help.

On-the-job productivity may also drop in a noisy environment, a number of studies suggest. In the most recent, 100 female college students were divided into two groups and placed in separate classrooms. They used computer terminals to take a standardized test much like the one given for admission to graduate school. The terminals in one room emitted a high-frequency tone that's produced by word processing equipment commonly found in offices and homes. The other monitors did not produce such a noise.

The noise-exposed women's overall productivity—based on their speed and accuracy on the test, among other measures—was about 8.5 percent lower than the control group's. The women with the noisy terminals worked at a faster pace, leaving them more prone to errors—an indication they were under stress.

"Women can hear higher-frequency ranges better than men," says Caroline Dow, Ph.D., assistant professor of communication at the University of Evansville in Indiana and one of the authors of the study. In fact, women are more sensitive than men in general to sound—they tend to become irritated by sounds at half the volume that men are. That may mean that women are more susceptible to noise-related health problems, researchers say.

Dr. Dow and her colleague also found that the noise-exposed women who were in the second or fourth week of their menstrual cycles scored even worse. "Women with high estrogen levels are even more sensitive to noise," Dr. Dow says.

This study measured the women's productivity only—it didn't look at their blood pressure levels or any other physical consequences. "But this type of stress can cause fatigue, jumpiness, irritation and persistent headaches," says study coauthor Douglas C. Covert, Ph.D., also an assistant professor of communication at the University of Evansville.

If you work with computers, you may be able to head off these potential problems by wearing earplugs, which can help reduce noise levels.

The Stress Connection

No one knows for sure how noise affects the interior workings of your body. But the most plausible theory to date is that it activates the "fight-or-flight" response— your body's typical reaction to any stressful situation.

"Sound can be perceived as aversive or painful," says Redford B. Williams, M.D., professor of psychiatry and director of the Behavioral Medicine Research Center at Duke University in Durham, North Carolina. "Your brain decides you're in an emergency situation and that you've got to fight it or flee. When this happens, adrenaline pours into your blood, and your nerves release norepinephrine—a type of hormone—throughout your body. That makes your heart beat faster and harder, pumping more blood to your muscles."

That's supposed to prime your muscles for a quick left jab or a quick exit. But if you sit there and steam over your neighbor's blaring stereo, the blood vessels in your muscles clamp down, resisting that extra flow. "That may, in theory, lead to high blood pressure," Dr. Williams says. "But if you used your muscles, that extra blood would be appropriate, and there wouldn't be that clamping down to keep the muscles from getting more blood than they need."

When you're ready to rumble or run, your mind can lose its focus, too. "Your body's telling you you're in danger, so you become more concerned with looking after yourself than with someone else's needs," Dr. Williams says. That may explain the irritability, aggressiveness, drops in productivity and learning impairment associated with noise.

The Annoyance Factor

Perception is a key word when you're talking about noise, because what's noise to you might be music to your neighbor. "If you're trying to get some work done in your office and there's a typewriter banging away outside the door, it makes a big difference if it's your secretary typing your stuff or your colleague's secretary typing his," says Jerome Singer, Ph.D., chairman of the Department of Medical Psychology at the Uniformed Services University of the Health Sciences in Bethesda, Maryland.

Whether or not a sound annoys you depends on a combination of factors besides its volume—the sound's pattern and purpose, among others. That means the noise may not have to be loud to set off your body's fight-or-flight reaction. The sporadically dripping faucet that keeps you up all night may register at 55 decibels or less—but it could be more annoying and thus more stress-producing than the 90 decibels of noise generated by a constant stream of traffic outside your office window. (The federal Occupational Safety and Health Administration mandates ear protection for workers exposed to noise at 89 decibels and above.)

The idea that everyday noise—like the whining dog next door or the buzz of the window fan at night—may cause health problems is intriguing. More research is needed to test its effects, though. Most of the studies done to date exposed subjects to sound at upwards of 85 decibels, four to eight hours a day, for months at a time—well above the levels you're likely to encounter.

Now, in Dr. Dow and Dr. Covert's study, the

244

computer tone wasn't ear-splitting. In fact, it ranged from about 42 to 49 decibels, similar to the level in an ordinary living room where you're having a conversation. The researchers say it was the frequency, not the volume, that caused the stress.

"If you perceive the noise as a stressor, you're going to trigger the release of stress hormones," Dr. Singer says. "But if you can control the sound or noise—or if it's predictable—it's not as threatening."

Dr. Peterson gave his noise-exposed monkeys an opportunity to reduce the volume of the noise during one of his experiments. Their blood pressures increased only one-third to one-half as much as the monkeys who didn't have control.

And in one experiment, Dr. Singer's subjects had the option of pushing a button to stop the noise if it was bothering them. "We told them that we preferred they didn't push it because we were trying to study the effects of noise," he says. "Even if they didn't push the button because they wanted to cooperate, having the button available reduced the physical effects. So if you think you can control it, you can moderate its effects."

Neutralize Noise with Soothing Sounds

There are some sounds you can't silence, like the roar of planes, trains and automobiles outside your bedroom window, the photocopy machines in the hall next to your office, the computer terminal you type on or the air-conditioning system's background buzz. You have to find some way to cope with them.

One strategy is to launch a counterattack with positive, stress-reducing sounds. "Sound can guide you to serenity, to become excited, to relieve that excitement—it's done in movies all the time," says psychotherapist and stress-management expert Emmett Miller, M.D., who for the last 20 years has produced relaxation tapes using music, natural sounds and his voice. "Smooth, flowing sounds train your body and mind to feel that way—smooth and flowing."

Sound has a direct effect on the hypothalmic area of your brain, Dr. Miller says, which influences the nerves, muscles and glands in your body and regulates your blood flow.

Here are the experts' suggestions for serene sounds that may head off high blood pressure and other ill effects of noise. What works for you is up to you, because everybody's definition of noise is different. So you may have to have several sound checks before you hit on the right one.

Use Instruments of Pleasure ▶ Research has suggested many possible benefits of music—it may lower heart rate and blood pressure, decrease anxiety and depression, relieve pain and increase feelings of well-being. In two studies, patients who listened to music

---

SOUNDPROOFING TIPS

Until research reveals more about whether noise can affect your health without damaging your hearing, the best way to protect yourself is to protect your ears. Here are some techniques for sound-proofing your life, straight from the experts.

Avoid it. Think about the noisemakers in your home and come up with alternatives. Consider discarding your blow-dryer and letting your hair dry naturally. Buy coffee that's already ground, instead of enduring the whir of an electric grinder. Make use of your knives instead of chopping vegetables in a food processor. Cut your grass with an old-fashioned push-mower. Beat your batter with a wooden spoon instead of an electric mixer. Retire your leaf blower and take up your rake.

Plug it. Earplugs offer quick and convenient protection from noise. According to researchers, plugs should be worn during high-noise activities, such as rock concerts or loud sporting events. You should also use them when operating power tools. Even vacuum cleaners and hair dryers can create enough noise to

before and during surgery had lower levels of stress hormones in their blood.

One of Dr. Miller's favorite antistress sounds is the shakuhachi, a kind of Japanese flute—but you may try the more traditional flute or flutelike instruments like the recorder. "Flutes glide between tones instead of playing one note after another," he says. "That produces a kind of wavelike feeling."

Steven Halpern, Ph.D., educator and composer, has found with biofeedback testing that people's stress levels tend to reduce when they listen to an electric piano. He also tried violin and oboe but found that they tended to irritate.

Dig Music with a Slow Beat ▶ Some music therapists speculate that tunes with tempos slightly slower

rattle your nerves. Cotton balls aren't good enough protection for your ears, either. You'd be better off getting a good pair of soft-foam plugs (available in drugstores for about $2). Check the label to make sure the earplugs you're buying reduce sound by at least 20 decibels, says noise researcher Ernest Peterson, Ph.D., of the University of Miami School of Medicine.

Turn it down. Most personal and car stereos have volume-control dials that go from 1 to 10. Keep yours set at 4 or below. If your stereo has a wider range, make sure you at least keep the volume at just under the midpoint or below.

Muffle it. Placing small appliances like blenders on rubber mats or stacks of dish towels can help reduce the racket in your home. Larger appliances, like washing machines, can also rest on rubber cushions to reduce noise-producing vibration.

Absorb it. Window drapes, carpeting and furniture soak up household sounds that tend to be amplified by bare walls and floors.

than your heart rate may slow your heart until it's in sync and cause short-term drops in blood pressure.

Try Easy-Listening Music ▶ In one study, treadmill joggers who listened to "elevator music" had lower heart rates and jogged longer than joggers who grooved to rock. Background music—in any setting—may take your attention off unpleasant noise. That's known as masking, a method used to treat tinnitus, which is characterized by a constant ringing in the ears.

Hear the Elements ▶ Listen to leaves rustling in a breeze, the rhythmic ebb and flow of the ocean or the rush of a good rain. "Nature's sounds tend to produce a consistent, pleasant background," Dr. Miller says. "There's a seeming randomness, but it's not really random. We can perceive a deeper structure if we just step back a little and listen with our 'third ear.' When we listen to the sounds of nature, I think we're picking up deeper, wavelike cycles that we cannot measure."

Of course, the real thing is usually best. But sometimes you need to hear the sounds of a storm when there's not a cloud in the sky. In that case, try the high-tech version—a "natural-sound" cassette tape or compact disc recording. Rainstorms, forest sounds complete with chirping birds, and ocean waves are among those available at most record stores.

Listen to the Sounds of Silence ▶ It used to be golden and now it's so rare it's positively platinum. But you can find silence in this noisy world—it just takes a little work. You can find it scuba diving in the sound-absorbing world of water, strolling in an evening snowfall or hiking through an isolated forest. You can seek out your own special quiet place in a neighborhood park, the local library—even create one in your own home.

But what about when you're harnessed to a computer eight hours a day, phones jingling, copiers clacking and air conditioners rumbling?

248

Try getting in touch with the silence within you through relaxation techniques or meditation. You can fix your mind on a sight, sound or smell that, in effect, blocks everything else out, and breathe slowly, in and out. "That won't control the stressor, but it controls your response to it, and thereby puts you in control," Dr. Williams says.

Friends for Life 29

Good relationships can make your life better and help you live longer.

Among the cacophony of "don'ts" and "do-not-evers" from the world of health and science comes a very happy "do"—as in duet—and it's this: Play together, be together, worry together, go to the doctor together, and all the while talk to each other in your daily rounds. It turns out that not only will your life be richer but you will probably live longer, as well.

According to a study at the Duke University Medical Center in Durham, North Carolina, simply having someone to talk to may be as important to your heart's health as costly medical treatment. The Duke research is based on a nine-year follow-up study of 1,368 patients initially admitted to Duke for cardiac catheterization to diagnose heart disease.

"We knew in exquisite detail how well their hearts functioned at the start of the study and, therefore, what their survival rates should have been," says Redford Williams, M.D., director of Duke's Behavioral Medicine Research Center and lead author of the study.

"What we found," he says, "was that those patients with neither a spouse nor a friend were three times more likely to die than those involved in a caring relationship."

After a heart attack, heart muscle damage is considered the number-one predictor of long-term survival, Dr. Williams explains. In this study, however, having a confidant or, conversely, being socially isolated, altered expected survival rates for better or worse.

For people with minimal heart muscle damage, for

example, the five-year death rate is about 10 percent. Of the patients with minimal heart muscle damage in the Duke study, however, just 5 percent of those with social support died. Meanwhile, 15 percent of the socially isolated patients died.

In patients with severe heart muscle damage, the results were even more dramatic. These people generally face about a 40 percent chance of dying within five years. But according to the Duke doctors, having friends cut the patients' risk to 20 percent, and lack of human companionship pushed it up to 60 percent.

Good Friends, Good Health

This isn't the first time research has demonstrated that good friends can be good medicine. For years, doctors have suspected a link. Then, in 1979, the so-called Alameda County Study made history with its nine-year follow-up findings on nearly 7,000 people (all of them residents of Alameda County, California).

What the researchers found was that, for every age group, there was a direct relationship between community or social ties and a person's chance of dying from any cause. People with the most social contacts were the least likely to die during the nine-year study period. Those who were the most isolated faced the greatest risk of dying. And these results were independent of traditional risk factors, such as smoking, excess body weight and lack of physical activity.

More recently, studies conducted in the United States (at Duke, Yale and Berkeley) and Europe have examined the role of social support on both healthy people and heart patients. The results are consistent: Socially isolated people (whether healthy or suffering from heart disease) were three to five times more likely to die than people with intimate relationships.

Intimate Details

Exactly what does a close friend bring to a patient's bedside? Researchers at Yale and the West Haven

Veterans Administration Medical Center who studied this matter offer a suggestion. The value of intimacy during recovery comes from the reassurance the patient gets that he is still valued in the eyes of his family, they say.

After a heart attack, for instance, a man in a hospital may worry that he won't be able to go back to work or be able to make love to his wife—that he will be unable to resume his place in his family. Although the stress from this is enormous, it can be ameliorated with love and understanding. In a supportive relationship, the healing process begins with the patient expressing fears and a loved one listening. The partner then can provide reassurance that the patient will indeed be a part of the family again. (Ideally, this point should be backed up by medical feedback from the patient's own doctors.) Patients receiving this type of support, studies conclude, do better and live longer than those without it.

In simple terms, what these patients feel is the security of being loved.

Feeling the security of a loving relationship is especially critical during the acute stages of an illness, such as the first few weeks or months following a heart attack. But the benefits go beyond the hospital bed. Several studies found that ongoing positive support improved patients' abilities to maintain healthier habits recommended by their doctors. That is, they were more likely to participate in hypertension control programs and stay away from cigarettes.

A Case in Point

These findings come as no surprise to Werner Hebenstreit of San Francisco. When he recently heard the results of the Duke study, he said grandly, "Well, of course."

Several years ago, at age 71, after two major heart attacks and two angioplasties (a procedure in which a small balloon is inflated inside a blood vessel), he thought he had little time left. That was before he agreed to participate in a research trial conducted by Dean Ornish, M.D., an assistant clinical professor of

251
■

medicine at the University of California and director of the Preventive Medicine Research Institute in Sausalito.

Dr. Ornish's program takes a total-lifestyle approach to treating heart disease. Patients are required to quit smoking, adopt a very low-fat diet, take a 45-minute walk every day and regularly practice some type of relaxation technique, such as meditation.

For many, these changes involve a 180-degree turn from their past. That's why Dr. Ornish insists that each patient's spouse or companion participate in the program, too—to provide much-needed support.

The first skill the couples learn together is communication. "Basic communication skills can be quite powerful in showing people how to increase the likelihood of surviving illness," says Dr. Ornish, author of *Dr. Dean Ornish's Program for Reversing Heart Disease.*

Werner Hebenstreit is a great example, Dr. Ornish explains, of how "the experience of transforming behaviors often can open up hearts in ways that go beyond unclogging arteries."

Werner remembers well the way he used to communicate. "I would come home from work and Eva, my wife, would say, 'How was your day?' and I would scream, 'I want to forget this day! Why do you want me to remember this day? This was a lousy day.'

"This," he says, chuckling at his past life, "is not talking." The Ornish program began with the couple on a week-long retreat, working on both communicating and exchanging feelings. "Now my relationship is wonderful," Werner exclaims. "We read and discuss books. We see and discuss films. If I have a lousy day, we sit down and we try to discover why it was lousy."

All that open communication has paid off in heart dividends, too. With Eva's support, Werner has persevered with the program and grown progressively healthier. Before beginning the program, two of his coronary arteries were more than 50 percent blocked and the third was totally clogged. But after four years on the program, the partially blocked arteries were just 13 percent closed, and the fully blocked artery had blood flowing through it.

Dr. Ornish agrees with the long-term care benefits cited in the Duke study and believes that it is the support of the friend or spouse that reinforces and perpetuates the change. In fact, he says, "It's very hard to get people to change their diets or stop smoking if they are not happy or supported."

New York newspaper columnist and Pulitzer Prize–winning war correspondent Sydney Schanberg knows this firsthand. Several years ago, he had a quadruple-bypass operation. Now, minus his cigars, butter and a few excess pounds, he says it is his very happy and healthy relationship with a special woman in his life that sustains him. That is true in no small part, Schanberg says, because "she participates in the lifestyle changes I must maintain to live."

The Health Connection

Without making the changes and having the support to maintain them, Dr. Ornish says, "bypasses just bypass the problem, and the symptoms and disease often return." The steps that create health-threatening stress now are understood by medical professionals, just as the path to recovery through communication can be measured.

It is our sense of isolation that initially disturbs us, according to Dr. Ornish. The fear that we cannot or should not reveal ourselves to others dislodges us from our more natural human feelings of connection, of being part of a tribe. It promotes discordant communication and leaves us isolated. That, in turn, leads to chronic stress.

"I don't think it's the fast pace of modern life," says Dr. Ornish, "but we previously were much more connected. One hundred years ago people had to worry that if it didn't rain the crops wouldn't come in and they'd starve. Clearly, that's at least as stressful as worrying whether your faxes came in."

But the disintegration of the extended family, Dr. Ornish believes, leaves us feeling somewhat addled and alone. Then our defenses come up. Those same defenses that protect us can isolate us and lead to a sense of vigilance.

"Chronic vigilance activates the 'fight-or-flight'

253

response," Dr. Ornish says. Chemically, the fight-or-flight response results in the excretion of chemicals in the body, including norepinephrine. "Although that is designed to protect us, when chronically turned on it harms us," Dr. Ornish explains. A study of people living near Pennsylvania's Three-Mile Island nuclear reactor a year after the accident, for example, found that those who felt more emotional support excreted less of these fight-or-flight chemicals.

Our sense of isolation may be reflected in how we sometimes defer happiness, believing that if we only had more money or more beauty or more accomplishments, we could be happy and people would like us. Not having these things can make us judge ourselves harshly and feel unlovable.

Sometimes, perhaps, we pretend to have something—some quality that sets us apart from others. But all the while we are vigilantly guarding against being found out—found out to be lacking in that very thing we think would make us special.

It's exhausting. And isolating.

Having someone to talk to gives us a safe place in which we can share what is going on in our lives. It helps us to get over that human fear that what we lack will always leave us lacking. It enables us to get past that so-typical fear: "If I tell you what I'm really like, you'll reject me," Dr. Ornish explains.

Instead, consider this: "If I tell you what I'm like, you might see I'm a lot like you." And that common bond might be the beginning of a great duet. Just letting down those walls and talking can be exquisitely healing.

Creating Harmony for Healing

Talking, it seems, may be good medicine for other illnesses, as well.

Studies have revealed positive relationships between social support and higher immune functions, low blood pressure and recovery from surgery.

Our goal, then, is harmony—to act and react with the people around us and to prevent or recover from the chronic illnesses stress can initiate. But in this world of people moving away from their families, traveling for jobs and going it solo, is all this easier said than done?

Dr. Williams doesn't think so.

"This social connection doesn't grow on trees, but we know it confers a benefit in all illnesses and in the prevention of illnesses," Dr. Williams says. "So even if you move away and live alone in a new community, getting connected should be a priority." Dr. Williams recommends first tapping whatever social support system you have—friends, neighbors, relatives. If you're new to a community, he suggests, join a religious or social group. If you already belong to a group, he says, increase your activity.

"What's important to your health and happiness is that the support system provides a forum where you can communicate," Dr. Williams says. "This gives you a group of people that you can share your feelings with. But it must be genuine. You have to invest to get something back."

In other words, friendship can be a prescription for health. So while some say talk is cheap, it's not. For our health, it's invaluable.

Return from Fear 30

People who fought their phobias—and won.

Few of us like to see a spider crawling down our wall. And most of us clench our teeth and start to sweat a little when an airplane ride turns bumpy.

But what if those natural fears became so intense that normal life became difficult or impossible? What if we fled in panic at the sight of any insect or refused to board an airplane, no matter what?

Then our fear would have crossed the line into phobia, says Anne Marie Albano, Ph.D., assistant director of the Center for Stress and Anxiety Disorders at the State University of New York at Albany. "A phobia is an unrealistic fear that is all out of proportion to the actual threat."

The fear of spiders, for instance, would be present even when there were no spiders around. "The most common fears people have are of animals or insects; natural elements like storms and water; and heights or closed-in spaces, like elevators. One traumatic event may trigger the phobia. An assault by one dog, for example, may lead to a fear of all dogs.

"No one knows for sure what causes phobias," says Dr. Albano. "But there's growing evidence that some people are genetically predisposed to them. If someone comes to the center with a phobia, we often find that another member of the family has a phobia, too."

Fortunately, phobias are very treatable, she says. "As many as 90 percent of people with phobias report recovery or significant progress after treatment."

Effective therapy focuses on relaxation, realistic thinking and gradual exposure to the source of the fear. People with mild phobias can successfully practice these techniques themselves with the aid of self-help groups and books. With more intractable phobias, just a few sessions with a skilled therapist can relieve the problem. If the phobia is very severe, lengthier and more intensive therapy may be needed.

The five people who tell their stories here triumphed over their phobias—living proof that it can be done.

Towering Terror

Twenty years ago, Jerilyn Ross was bewildered by her irrational fear of going up in tall buildings. Today, at 45, as head of the Anxiety Disorders Association of America (ADAA) and director of the Ross Center for Anxiety and Related Disorders in Washington, D.C., she understands. This is her story:

"It started on a wonderful summer night when I was 25. I was having a great time traveling in Europe with a girlfriend. On that particular evening, we were in Salzburg, Austria, in a dramatically lovely restaurant. The building was set high up on the side of a mountain. The dance floor was huge and slightly sloped, leading to large glass windows and a balcony overlooking the town.

"A handsome man asked me to dance. The lights of Salzburg were glittering as we spun around the floor. I was ecstatic. I remember thinking, 'This is the most beautiful place I've ever been.'

"Suddenly, out of nowhere, I had this overpowering fear that I might run to the edge of the building and jump off the balcony. It was the most frightening feeling of my life.

"I didn't know what to do, so I excused myself abruptly, grabbed my girlfriend and ran down the stairs. I never went back or saw my handsome prince again.

"When I returned home to Manhattan, my life changed completely. For the next five years, I avoided going above the tenth floor of any building. I don't know why the tenth and not the ninth floor, but that was it.

"I couldn't understand what had happened. I'd had a very happy childhood; I'd never been depressed, and certainly I wasn't suicidal. I was working successfully as a grade-school math teacher. I felt my life was wonderful in every way, and yet the terror was so overwhelming.

"Every time my phone rang, I was afraid I'd have to go up a high building. The worst was having to manipulate friends: They'd call and say, 'Let's have dinner on top of the World Trade Center,' and I'd say, 'Oh, I ate there last week. The food isn't very good. Why don't you come over here?' I became a great cook.

"What was strange was that before and after the phobia began, I was an avid skier: I skied on glaciers and rode high mountain gondolas with no problem with heights.

"While I was teaching, I was attending graduate school at night in psychology. I'd spend hours in the library trying to diagnose the problem I was experiencing. I couldn't find an explanation. I was convinced I had some strange disorder that no one else had or ever heard of.

"No one knew about my fear, except the girlfriend I

257

traveled with and a psychoanalyst I dated at the time. He'd say, 'You just think you had a good childhood. This indicates some awful thing that you've repressed, and you ought to get into analysis.' That made me feel even worse.

"Finally, in 1978, I read a magazine article about a hospital-run therapy group for people with all these strange fears, like a lawyer who couldn't go on subways. They were like me—normal, healthy people with weird thoughts. I signed up with the group immediately.

"Meeting others helped, but what really changed things was when the therapist took me by the hand into tall buildings. We took small steps at first. I'd go up and down a few more stories each time.

"Every time I'd start to panic, the therapist would say, 'Stay with the feeling; it will pass,' and it did. I learned I could face down my fear.

"After just a few weeks, I made it above the tenth floor. For 'graduation' after 12 weeks, my assignment was to have a drink on the top of the Gulf & Western Building, 44 awful stories high. Reaching the top took so much out of me that I felt like I'd just won an Olympic medal. I was wiped out but happy.

"Now, as director of my own treatment center for phobias and other anxiety disorders, I take other people up buildings. I tell people I'm not completely cured, just like someone might say he's an alcoholic even though he hasn't had a drink in 20 years. But I don't avoid anything anymore. When I go to hotels and they say the penthouse is available, I take it—just for practice.

"I have a better understanding of my phobia now. It may run in my family: When I finally told my mother about my problem, she told me she'd had phobias. I also think I know why the first panic attack hit on that evening in Salzburg. I think it was the overwhelming beauty of that night: the glistening lights, the castles twinkling, the handsome guy dancing and spinning me around. There was too much stimulation: The body doesn't know the difference between good stress and bad stress.

258

"About three years ago, while I was in Austria for a ski trip, I felt I had to go back to that restaurant in Salzburg. I spent two hours walking around the town, summoning my courage to go into the building and up to the rooftop restaurant. Finally I made the move and went up.

"The room didn't look anywhere near as scary as I'd remembered, nor did it seem as high. It was small and closed in, and the floor wasn't nearly as tilted toward the windows as I recalled. I wanted to ask someone if they'd renovated, but no one spoke English. So I took a seat right up against the windows, and I sat there for an hour, crying and trying to write in my diary.

"I wasn't crying because I was afraid; I felt no fear there at all. I was crying because this was where it all started. I realized I had turned it all around and was now able to help other people do the same."

Bridge to Freedom

For Ron Bednar, 46, who directs purchasing for a hospital located in the San Francisco area, the region's most famous landmark was once his worst nightmare. His story:

"A few years ago, I was working as a free-lance artist. From where I live—about 15 miles north of San Francisco—I had to cross the Golden Gate Bridge to get to the city, where most of the jobs were. The problem was, I had an incredible amount of trouble driving across bridges. I'd have full-blown panic attacks—sweating, shaking—it was an awful feeling. Like I was dying. And I would do anything to avoid that feeling again.

"So frequently I would turn down work in San Francisco. I'd take buses. Or I'd convince a friend to drive me. I was fine if someone else was driving. Occasionally, I could white-knuckle it across the Golden Gate alone, all the while thinking, 'There must be something wrong with me.' My world became smaller.

"The bridge phobia was the tip of the iceberg. Since childhood, I'd experienced fears, particularly fears of leaving a safe place. They'd show up under periods of severe stress.

"The low point came one Christmas 12 years ago, when my son was five. I was to meet him at his grand-

259
∎

parents' house on Christmas morning, in San Francisco. As I approached the Golden Gate I had this incredible feeling of doom and terror.

"I turned around and went home. I didn't spend that Christmas with my son. And I felt horrible for years about missing that day with him. Then I heard about a therapist who specializes in phobias, Victoria Johnson, Psy.D., director of the Phobia Center in Marin County, California. She offered a 12-week group program; I signed up.

THREE STEPS TO STOP THE FEAR

Effective phobia fighting usually takes a combination of the following three techniques. If your phobia is mild, you may even be able to use these techniques to overcome it on your own.

The calming breath. Relaxation techniques, such as meditating, deep-breathing exercises or listening to relaxation tapes can help defuse panic in a frightening situation. Here's how to practice what's known as the calming breath.

• Take in a long, slow breath through your nose, first filling your lower lungs, then your upper lungs.

• Hold your breath to the count of three. Then exhale through pursed lips, while you relax the muscles in the face, jaws, shoulders and stomach.

• Practice this several times a day or when the going gets rough.

Cognitive therapy. This sophisticated version of positive thinking is a proven way to block fear. Most phobics get caught up in irrational, negative thinking that scares them more: "What if that dog bites me?" That's why it's important to recognize negative thoughts by writing them down on a small pad that you carry with you. Then, come up with realistic, positive thoughts to substitute: "That dog never bit anyone." You may need to do some research to come up with realistic substitutes. Erstwhile fearful-flyer Barbara Katz, a social worker from Boston, was helped by facts about the rarity of airplane crashes.

"It started out like a college class. She explained what phobias are. I learned that phobics are masters of visualization, but what we visualize are catastrophes. For example, I'd drive down the road thinking, 'Gee, I feel a little nervous. What if I get so nervous I can't drive? What if I crash? What if I go crazy and jump off?' It would spiral to the point where I was hyperventilating, sweating and shaking.

"I learned to replace catastrophic thinking with posi-

Behavioral therapy. Once people have learned relaxation techniques and are able to use realistic thoughts to replace the frightening ones, they're ready to begin a type of behavioral therapy called gradual desensitization. It means, simply, facing the things they fear.

"We arrange for people to confront the object in a way that the fear won't be overwhelming. But it will be strong enough that they learn they can overcome it," says David Barlow, Ph.D., director of the Center for Stress and Anxiety Disorders at the State University of New York at Albany.

Start by confronting a version of your feared object that's just a little bit scary, says Dr. Barlow. "For example, if the feared object is an insect, we might start by showing them a picture of it. Then we try to capture the insect and keep it in a glass aquarium across the room. Then they have to get near it. We practice each level until they're comfortable."

For a list of therapists and support groups, contact the Anxiety Disorders Association of America (ADAA). This national nonprofit organization offers a directory with the names of more than 700 specialists who treat phobias and panic disorders, along with a list of self-help organizations and information on phobias and other anxiety disorders. Send $3 to ADAA, 6000 Executive Bldg., Suite 513, Rockville, MD 20852.

261

tive thoughts: 'I drive extremely well even when I'm anxious.' Dr. Johnson says that in 14 years of working with phobias, she has never heard of anyone with a driving phobia who had an accident because of it. Something else she told me really helped: 'Drive the road, not your emotions.'

"I learned to block the physical fear, too. Did my chest feel tight? I'd take a deep breath and relax. Was I gripping the wheel too tightly? I'd relax my hands. Was I staring straight ahead, too scared to look left or right? I'd deliberately scan the road from side to side. I practiced diaphragmatic breathing—long, deep, relaxing breaths. Regular exercise was a big help; while I was recovering, I'd do 20 minutes twice a day of cardiovascular aerobic exercise.

"After several weeks of classroom learning, we started field work. First, I'd drive toward the bridge and park, then walk a ways to look at it. Later, I walked up to it and touched it. The next step was to walk a little way on it. The day finally came when I walked across the entire bridge. I was scared when I got out in the middle. But now I understood my fear, and I knew I had the tools to change it.

"The next challenge was driving onto and across the bridge. People in the class helped me. They'd sit in the back seat while I drove.

"There was no blinding flash of light; the fear just gradually dropped away. One day I had some business in San Francisco. I got in the car and decided I was going and that was it. I drove across the bridge, did my work, and drove back. I had finally reached the point where I could take care of what needed to be done. I wasn't afraid anymore."

Things That Go Bump

Animal fears are the most common simple phobia. Fears like these hardly threaten the livelihoods of most people. But even a mild animal phobia can be a real problem if you're a veterinarian, says Bart Iaia, D.V.M., 27, a graduate of the Tufts University School of Veterinary Medicine. Here's what happened with her:

"I went into veterinary medicine because I really liked dogs and cats. And I liked farm animals, too. I spent a year working on a farm in Scotland and handled sheep and pigs with no problem.

"But I was always uncomfortable around reptiles, such as snakes and other things that go bump in the night. That fear started when I was a child. A friend of mine invited me over to see his new pet. He brought me to his closet and opened the door. Out jumped a hissing, three-foot-long iguana. It didn't really bite or attack, but I was terrified.

"Years later, when I decided to go into veterinary medicine, that iguana was in the back of my mind. I knew that one day I'd be sitting in my office and someone would come in with a weird reptile—one that I'd have to deal with. I didn't know if I could.

"I came face-to-face with my fear the day I walked into the exotic-animal clinic at veterinary school for a two-week rotation. I looked around at all the reptiles and said to myself, 'If it doesn't have hair, I don't want to handle it.'

"The first few days of that rotation were really tough. But I guess just being around all those snakes and lizards for hours on end operated like its own desensitization program, because the edge of my fear was gradually blunted. My stint at the exotic-animal clinic actually ended up being a blessing in disguise.

"I started watching the veterinarians carefully to see how they handled the animals. I asked a lot of questions. They gave me accurate, useful information that replaced my frightening thoughts. Instead of thinking, 'This snake could attack me,' I would think, 'We've lowered the room temperature, which slows snakes down so they can be controlled more easily.' Facts replaced fears.

"The more time I spent with them and the more I learned, the more comfortable I became.

"Then one day, someone brought in an iguana—my original nightmare. But I forced myself to look more closely at the animal, and I realized it was a very small, very sick little iguana. What possible threat could it be

263

to me? So I was able to handle it. I can't say I liked the feel of that scaly skin, but that moment really broke the back of my fear.

"Now I feel like I can handle anything, whether it has hair or not.

"And I think I'm better prepared to deal with clients who have animal fears. If a parent comes to me and says, 'Johnny wants to bring home a snake, and I'm scared,' I know what to say. 'First,' I tell them, 'go to a zoo and just spend a little time watching the snakes. Give yourself a reward for doing it. Then read some books about snakes. Then have your child introduce you to some snakes. Work your way up slowly and gradually. Eventually, you'll become less and less afraid. It worked for me.'"

Red Flag

Injections, violent movies and the sight of blood make many people queasy. But for some, the problem gets out of hand. It's called a "blood and injury phobia." Blood and injury phobia is a little different, though. Like other phobic reactions, it starts with a rapid rise in heart rate. But then blood pressure and heart rate drop dramatically, and the person usually faints.

Sarah McKinley, 17, a high school senior, faced down a severe phobia of this kind with the help of the staff of the Center for Stress and Anxiety Disorders at the State University of New York at Albany. (We've changed Sarah's name.)

Although Sarah was young, the sudden onset of her phobia is exactly like that of many older adults, notes the center's Dr. Albano. "It even happens in physicians, who after years of treating injuries suddenly start fainting at the sight of them."

This is Sarah's story:

"In grammar school, if we had to watch a gory film, I closed my eyes during the bloody parts. That wasn't unusual; everyone else did the same thing as I did.

"But then, one day about a year ago, I was sitting in homeroom, reading a newspaper, when I saw a photograph of bloody palm prints on a wall. I looked at it and passed out. That was the first time.

"The school sent me home. I knew that looking at the photograph had completely grossed me out, but I didn't worry about it too much.

"Then came a sort of turning point. In a social studies class, they showed us an incredibly bloody movie about the Civil War. A soldier was blown up, and I fainted right there.

"After that I started fainting about once a week. Then twice a week, then every day, then four or five times a day. The Gulf War was going on at that time, so magazines and newspapers were full of bloody images and ideas. In English class, we'd read stories in which people were injured, and those scared me. In biology class, talking about body parts made me faint. I think my imagination was too vivid. My mom and I drove by an auto accident once, and even though I couldn't see the injuries, I imagined them and fainted. I couldn't look at any kind of raw meat.

"It got so bad that when a teacher handed me back a math test with corrections written in red ink, I thought of blood. The next thing I knew, I was lying on the ground.

"No one was really sure what was going on. Early on, I was brought to an emergency room. What a fiasco. The guy kept asking me if I was pregnant! Then he decided there was nothing wrong with me. Another doctor told my parents I'd have to be on medications for the rest of my life.

"We went to a neurologist, and he said my brain was fine. He said I needed to see a psychologist, that what I actually had was a phobia. My parents found the Center for Stress and Anxiety Disorders.

"They asked me to write out a hierarchy, starting with the situation I found least anxiety provoking and working all the way up to the scariest. At the bottom of my list I wrote down things like, 'looking at a Band-Aid' and 'seeing something red.' At the top, the most scary things I listed were 'seeing someone bleeding,' and 'watching a gory movie.'

"The psychologists told me that most people with phobias must be taught to relax in scary situations. But people who faint need to learn the opposite response:

265
∎

how to tense up our bodies and keep them tense, so our blood pressure doesn't drop and we don't pass out.

"First I practiced tensing and holding with separate muscle groups, like the hands, the arms and the legs. Then I learned to tense and hold all the muscles at the same time. I learned to do it sitting, standing up—in a variety of positions.

"Then the therapists asked me to choose music that made me feel cheerful. I picked Billy Joel music and brought in my favorite tape. That's when we were ready to start working on the hierarchy list.

"At first I had to write the word *blood* over and over again. I'd tense all my muscles, and sometimes they'd play the Billy Joel music that I liked. We'd do that until I was completely comfortable writing *blood* and then move up to the next level. They'd bring in pieces of raw meat, scary pictures, gory movies. I'd tense and listen to the music.

"By the end of about three months, I wasn't fainting anymore and could do all the things on my hierarchy without feeling nervous.

"My final tasks were to have my blood drawn and to watch a hip operation. And I actually found the hip operation interesting. I think the therapist who came along with me was more upset than I was. He'd never seen an operation, and I noticed he kept his arms folded, which is one way of doing the tension exercise without anyone knowing.

"I'll probably always be a little bit squeamish about blood and injuries. But nowadays, it's no big deal."

Fear of Flying

For people who fear flying, information about aviation can be a big help. Just ask Boston social worker Barbara Katz:

"I don't think I was afraid of flying as a young adult. It started in my thirties, and the fear came from my mother. She was terrified of flying—she never flew until the last ten years of her life. And she was convinced that if I got on an airplane, it would crash.

"Her pressure on me was worst when my children were young. If I told her I was flying somewhere, she told me I was an awful mother. How could I think about flying? My children were going to be orphans! We actually knew someone who was killed in an airplane crash, and she'd say, 'Don't you remember what happened to him?'

"It started to get to me. I remember once, driving on a highway in Boston toward the airport with tears streaming down my face, because we were going to fly to New Orleans, and that meant I was a terrible mother.

"When I did get on an airplane to go somewhere, I'd be incredibly nervous. I started making excuses for not flying. I didn't have to travel much for my job, but my husband traveled a lot for his, and I had opportunities to go with him. He'd be going someplace exciting, and I'd make a flimsy excuse for not going.

"One day my husband told me that he had to go on an extended trip to California. It sounded wonderful and I really wanted to go! But I just couldn't face getting on an airplane. I invented yet another excuse. That's when I really recognized what was going on, and I didn't like it. A friend told me about a local class for fearful flyers, held at the airport and taught by a psychologist. My friend and I enrolled in it together.

"They taught us relaxation exercises as well as why things happen on an airplane. I always disliked the smell of gasoline on planes when you'd first get on—I thought it meant something was wrong—but I learned that it's normal. I learned that turbulence doesn't mean the plane is falling apart. I learned that the air is calmer in the early morning, so that's a good time to fly. Also, sitting in the back of the airplane is a rougher ride than up front, in front of the wings. They even told us just how much of an airplane could be out of commission and it would still be able to land. I found it very, very interesting.

"The course was 15 years ago, but I still use the information that I learned there: It works. In the past three months, I traveled to Florida and Denver; in two weeks I'm going to Washington and after that to Oklahoma. Nowadays, if I turn down a trip, it's because I really can't go!"

Young
for
Life

**Breakthrough products to help
keep your skin moist and pliable.**

The main job of moisturizers has been to prevent moisture loss. But here are some of the benefits cosmetic scientists hope to perfect in the next ten years.

■ Products that are a more effective moisture barrier and boost the skin's natural sun-protection ability.

■ Products that can synthetically recondition the material that bonds the living skin cells together.

■ Ingredients that will help speed up cell regeneration.

■ Technology that will also make sure these new ingredients penetrate to the level of your skin where they'll do the most good.

"One problem has been to enable the skin's dead, dry upper layer to retain moisture," explains Charles Fox, cosmetic scientist and independent consultant to the cosmetics industry. "The first challenge is to develop the perfect barrier—a waterproof material that can hold moisture in and also soften the stiff stratum corneum."

Keeping Moisture In

"Cosmetic science is coming to understand what happens physiologically when a moisturizer interacts with the skin," says Edward M. Jackson, Ph.D., director of product integrity for the Andrew Jergens Company "This knowledge is enabling us to duplicate and enhance the materials involved in the process."

"It was thought that water was the only thing that could soften skin and that it was the key ingredient in a moisturizer," says Fox. "Now we've found that other materials can do the same thing better because they also help hold water. There are water-insoluble ingredients like lipids that are more important in terms of the interaction of the skin with water."

Lipids are the mortar holding the living skin cells together. They're fatty materials that attract, hold and then redistribute the moisture in your skin.

Your skin is constantly losing lipids. "It's not just mature skin that has lower lipid levels—young people lose lipids because they wash so frequently that they remove them faster than their bodies can manufacture them," says Dr. Jackson.

New and Improved Moisturizers

Lipids are one of the booming areas of cosmetic science. Research is going on in the three major types of intercellular lipids: fatty acids (petrolatum), ceramides and the cholesterols.

"For instance, right now at Jergens, we're very interested in the skin's intercellular lipids," says Dr. Jackson. "We're excited about the third family (the cholesterols), especially one of its members, cholesteril isostearate, which is in our Jergens Advanced Therapy lotions.

"Just as in the pharmaceutical world scientists translate knowledge of how the body works into synthetic drugs—like insulin—that can perform the same function as body systems, we've refined synthetic lipid analogs to mimic the normal materials that are present in healthy skin."

"Our top antiaging moisturizers, Ceramide Time Complex moisture creme and Ceramide Time Complex capsules, today incorporate members of the ceramide family of lipids," says John McCook, vice president of research and development at Elizabeth Arden. "Ceramides are lipids that help repair the barrier function of the skin so that it can retain moisture, which in turn keeps it flexible and elastic. We and other researchers have found that if you combine ceramide with certain other lipid molecules, you can boost the barrier repair process. Without this, using a moisturizer is like having the air conditioner on in the summer and having your window open. It's a wasted effort."

Moisturizers containing cholesteril isostearate and ceramides are at your drug or department store today. Other new ingredients to look for on your moisturizer label include alpha hydroxy acids, glycolic acid and hyaluronic acid. Meanwhile, it will take more studies to determine which of these ingredients—or which combination of ingredients—is the most beneficial moisturizer.

Environmental Protection

"We think that the ceramides in our products help protect against chemical pollutants in the air," says McCook. "It's also important to keep the number of ingredients that might be irritants, like preservatives, to a minimum. We already offer part of our ceramides line in capsules that contain no preservatives. They're as pure as we can make them."

"The most important thing you can do for your skin is to protect it from the sun," says Nicholas J. Lowe, M.D., clinical professor of dermatology at the University of California, Los Angeles, School of Medicine. "For this reason many skin-care companies have added sunscreens to their moisturizers. There's still room for improvement in the sunscreens themselves, however, and this is where the research on vitamin C as a sunscreen that also helps to repair sun damage may prove valuable."

Cosmeceuticals

The word *cosmeceutical* refers to materials that cross the line between cosmetics and drugs. One example is Retin-A. While it was used originally as an antiacne medication, patients who tried it also noticed an overall improvement in minor wrinkling and age spots. Albert Kligman, M.D., professor of dermatology at the University of Pennsylvania in Philadelphia, began using Retin-A on some patients to treat wrinkles, and it was shown to have cosmetic applications.

271

Retin-A also typifies the major stumbling block new

moisturizing ingredients face. As soon as a company claims their material actually changes the physiology of the skin (as opposed to just its appearance), it must be considered a drug and undergo costly, lengthy and necessary testing. Even Retin-A, which already has Food and Drug Administration approval as an antiacne medication, has to reapply for approval as a wrinkle treatment.

32 Shake a Leg

Country-western dancing is sweeping the country; even the guys are showing up.

You have to go see country-western dancing in action to know how much fun people are having. And when, during a line dance (no partner needed), you see more men on the dance floor than women, you know there's something happening with the potential to sweep the entire country.

Many men have never really been comfortable with freestyle, expressionistic dancing. Women often take to the dance floor alone or with other women. The females have fun gyrating and bouncing to the beat while the guys stand on the sidelines—or dance half-heartedly and self-consciously.

With the return of big-band dancing, women have coaxed their men to classes, hoping they can enjoy partner dancing. But some men are intimidated by the rigors of leading and find the dress codes of the ballroom stuffy.

"The guys seem to like the ambience of country-western dancing," says Beverly Ott, country-western teacher at the Midnight Rose nightclub in Quakertown, Pennsylvania. "There are rules to follow, which makes them feel more secure. They can memorize the steps for whole dances. The dance steps are choreographed, and both the man and the woman know what to do next.

That takes a lot of pressure off the guy."

The result is, in many parts of the country, you can go country-western dancing or take lessons seven nights a week! And as lessons and country-western dance halls proliferate, more people switch to country-western dancing because they can always find a place to go.

That Down-Home Feeling

So what is the ambience of country-western dancing? First of all, the dress is relaxed. Jeans, T-shirts and smooth-soled shoes are acceptable. After you become dedicated to the dance style, you can buy your cowboy hat, cowboy boots, fancy shirt, bolo tie and silver belt buckle. Think about it! What American boy has not dreamed of being a cowboy? And don't forget the cowgirls! The women wear full, swirling skirts with lace trim, or fringe that sways one way while they sway the other.

The atmosphere is friendly. Since everyone is dressed down in jeans or dressed up in country-western duds, there's no telling if you're a doctor or a truck driver.

"It's not true that country-western dancers are primarily blue collar," says Nancey Sheppard, owner of Satin 'n Denim dance studio in Media, Pennsylvania. "My students come from all walks of life. And they are warmer and more accepting of every way of life than any other dance group I've experienced. Country-western is a dance style that transcends culture and status. Once you put on your country clothes, nobody knows what you do for a living. And nobody cares. There's probably a lot of stress release just in that factor."

The Rise of the Urban Cowboy

Country-western dancing is a relative newcomer to the dance world. Although the partner dances borrow strongly from ballroom and polka traditions (there are country waltzes, polkas and jitterbugs), the unique style that's country-western was glamorized in 1978 by John Travolta and the movie *Urban Cowboy*. Disco dancing was dying, and the clubs were looking for a new fad.

That movie glorified the country-western dance halls of Houston.

And slowly but surely, the fad caught on, spreading outward to California and then across to the East. A dozen years later, cities in New Jersey, New York, Pennsylvania and Connecticut had more cowboys and cowgirls than the Wild West ever did.

The Midnight Rose is a case in point. A year ago, business in the sports bar was dwindling, according to owner Joe Gentile. On a whim, he suggested to his brother, who manages the club, that he try a country-

BOOTS AND STUFF

Just so you know, cowboys do not remove their hats when they enter a building. If you feel silly driving around in your car with yours on, wait till you get to the country-western dance. Plenty of men will be wearing them, and your self-consciousness will evaporate.

The same with boots. While any smooth-soled shoe is good for country dancing, only beginners come without their cowboy boots. Boots come in many colors and styles. Women seem to prefer white, but red, blue, brown and black are not uncommon. Real dance boots have suede soles that shouldn't be worn on the street. To protect your feet and lower back, heels should be no more than one inch high.

If you're interested in fancy country clothing or boots and you don't know where to go shopping, look for a tack shop. They sell riding gear as well as boots and hats. Other shops, called western shops, are completely devoted to outfitting country dancers. Ask people who wear outfits you like. They may know of a good mail-order business or a seamstress who custom-makes matching outfits. Women love the full, swirling skirts. They make turns and twirls beautiful to look at. And they feel great.

western band. "The next time I saw him, he was exhausted from staying up late, taking care of the country-western crowd. We expanded the dance floor three times in the last year to accommodate more dancers. We have a springboarded dance floor, which means the floorboards are resting on four-by-eights. This creates a resonating space so that when dancers stomp, they get a satisfying, booming sound. People come from all over to dance here now. We've got the largest country-western dance floor in Pennsylvania. And we give lessons for a nominal charge."

Texas Two-Step to Cotton-Eyed Joe

The accessibility of lessons is probably a major reason country-western dance is spreading so quickly. Unlike ballroom studios, where lesson contracts may cost hundreds of dollars, country-western teachers teach in nightclubs, often at the expense of the management rather than the students. Or you can sign up for a six- or eight-week series of lessons at churches, YMCAs or social halls for very reasonable fees.

Check the announcements or ads in a local newspaper for nightclubs that offer free lessons. Or call the local recreation board or YMCA.

The best way to find a class is by word of mouth. People can tell you how well a teacher handles a class and if he or she goes slowly enough for everyone to get it right.

Teachers are coordinating their efforts to standardize teaching so that a Cotton-Eyed Joe line dance in Pennsylvania is the same as the one they're doing in Los Angeles.

The National Teachers Association, based in Las Vegas, is a national group of country-western teachers helping each other develop a uniformity to their craft. President Kelly Gellette has written many step-by-step books for teachers and students. And a yearly directory is published, listing country-western dance teachers.

"For us, Kelly's books were our only resource for learning to dance," says Gerry Jines, a country-western teacher in Reading, Pennsylvania. "And if I got confused, I'd call her and ask her questions."

A very safe, nonthreatening way to get a glimpse of country-western dancing is on TV. Remember "American Bandstand"? Cable-TV viewers can turn to the Nashville channel in the late afternoon and get the country-western version, "Club Dance." (Check with your local cable company or television guide for times.) This is just what the crowd might look like in your neck of the woods: just social dancers having a good time.

If you want to perfect your styling and perhaps try competitive dancing, there are country-western dance studios where you can get private lessons. "You don't have to sign up for elaborate contracts," says Kristin Marstiller, owner of the Kactus Rose dance studio in Laurel, Maryland. "Most country-western studios contract by the hour."

Line Dancing

When people who are used to freestyle dancing go to a country-western bar for the first time, they often feel a little frustrated. Although the atmosphere is casual, lessons are as necessary in country-western as they are in ballroom dancing.

"You're not able to jump on the floor and move and shake to your own beat," says Sheppard. "Country-western dancing is a dance of community. And that's what a lot of people are looking for these days."

If you're venturing into country-western dancing on your own, try to find a class that specializes in line dancing. In line dancing, men stand with their thumbs in their belt loops or pockets. Women place their hands on their hips or use them expressively. The upper body is held straight. All the work is from the waist down. Moves like grapevines, shuffles, kicks, pivots, cha-cha steps and stomps are put together in varying combinations to accompany certain types of songs. Often a line dance matches a specific song, like the recently popular Achy Breaky Heart dance.

276

"Once you get a repertoire of steps under your belt, you often find that you can pick up the line dances much more quickly," says Marstiller, who is also a member of the United Country Western Dance Council.

You repeat a sequence of steps, which may be 16 counts or up to 180 counts (the average is about 56). Then you repeat the sequence until the music ends. Everyone moves together, as they do in synchronized swimming. People who are very comfortable with the steps may add some distinctive, individual styling. No two people wiggle alike. You'll find names like Tush Push, Boot Scootin' Boogie and County Line dance. Many enthusiasts dance several times a week and know as many as 100 line dances!

Be sure to stand tall and be conscious of your posture. "Good posture is essential," says Sheppard. "At first, dancing all weekend left me with back pain during the week. But working on correct posture eliminated it. Stand tall. Roll your shoulders, bring them up and down. Don't slump. You'll look better and feel better."

Partner Dancing

The Texas Two-Step is probably the best-known and easiest-to-learn country-western partner dance. Couples dance side by side or facing each other, with one partner moving backward. Dancers form a large circle on the perimeter of the dance floor and move counterclockwise around the floor. Slower dancers take the inside lane, faster dancers the outside lane. Men, for the most part, keep moving forward as they twirl the women in turns.

Waltz is also popular but moves in the line of dance, too, rather than as a box step in small circles. And there are polkas, cha-chas and swing dances, too.

Some partner dances are completely choreographed, and the partners perform the series of steps together, then repeat. Again, the circle is formed and all dancers move together in the line of dance. Sometimes singles join the circle and walk through the steps alone. Or two women dance side by side, without holding hands.

Here's a little tip for newcomers on styling. Men, place your right arm under the lady's left arm, with your right arm around her back at her left shoulder blade. Women, your left elbow should be nestled on top of the man's right elbow, with your hand on the front of his right shoulder. Your elbows should form a hinge. It may feel strange at first, but you'll fit right into the country crowd!

Dance-Floor Etiquette

Sound like there's a whole bunch going on? There is! And here's what you need to know to have fun and avoid crashes or sitting out when you could be dancing.

A good country-western dance floor is big enough to accommodate line dancers and partner dancers at the same time. A great floor also has room for swing and

HE OVERCAME SELF-CONSCIOUSNESS; SHE STIFLED ARTHRITIS

John Harvey and Carol Salvatore first saw country-western dancing at a "Country Night" on a cruise. Carol loved it. When a friend back home asked her to come to a group lesson, she begged John to join her. "He hated it," says Carol. "He'd make one mistake and feel everyone was watching him. He'd stand by the piano the rest of the night and refuse to even try. He was nicknamed 'the piano man' by the teachers.

"Believe it or not, I talked him into two more sets of lessons. We enjoyed the people we met, and he liked the music. I especially loved the dancing. It wasn't until the third six-week session that he finally started to relax and learn.

"He's a truck driver, and now when he travels he looks for the closest place to dance every night. He's been in nightclubs all up and down the East Coast. He'll take whatever lesson they have to offer. There is always something new to learn."

Joan Messina took up country-western dancing after her husband passed away some years back.

"I was depressed, and my arthritis was very painful," she says. "A friend invited me to a line-dance

freestyle dancing. Dance-floor etiquette is important for ease of dancing and everyone's enjoyment. Line dancers head for the center of the room. Swing and freestyle dancers can find a space alongside them if there's room. Although in reality, line dances are often so popular, freestylers and swing dancers may get crowded off the floor. Technically, it's fair for you to demand your space. Practically speaking, most people join the crowd or sit down.

There are almost always two-steppers dancing around the perimeter, in fast and slow lanes. You can't stop and chat on the dance floor. You would create a major traffic jam and be very unpopular. If you get

---

class, and I liked it. It was good to get out and move. We started practicing in her basement, and her husband got interested in dancing, too. He found a partner for me, and we all started going to lessons together.

"My depression lifted, and I found that the dancing kept me limber. There are some nights I feel I might be too stiff and sore to dance, but I just take a hot shower, put on my boots and go. As soon as the music starts, I'm on the floor, and as far as I'm concerned, the pain is gone.

"I usually feel wonderful the next day. Sure, if I dance for five or six hours straight, my feet might be sore. Whose wouldn't? If I miss dancing for a week or more, my body stiffens right up. I used to walk regularly to stay limber, but now I dance almost every day instead. I love it because dancing is a social as well as an exercise activity. It's helped me keep off the 50 pounds I lost by dieting, too."

Joan hand-paints her own country-western clothing, which also helps keep her arthritic hands flexible. "It's opened up a whole new world for me," she says.

confused or lose your step, move toward the center and give dancers a passing lane to get around you.

If you're a beginner and two-step is all you know, don't be shy around the line dancers. Get up there and two-step to your heart's content around them. You're not out of place or doing anything odd. Don't be surprised if other couples follow your lead.

33   Whole-Body Healing

Yoga stretches the body, mind and spirit.

At first glance, a yoga class looks like any aerobic dance workout. Students in leotards or sweat suits distribute themselves around a large open room and unroll exercise mats. The teacher greets them and says, "Let's begin."

But unlike aerobics, jazzercize or any of today's other dance-for-fitness programs, yoga classes involve neither loud music nor high-stepping cheerleader-style routines. Instead the room stays quiet and the participants remain relatively still as the teacher leads them in a 60- to 90-minute series of stretches that resemble the neck rolls, hip twists, hurdler's stretches and other warm-up exercises athletes do before games or races.

But on closer inspection, yoga stretches are different from other sports' warm-ups.

Yoga Is Slower ▶ Students might take as long as a minute to ease into stretched postures, and then hold them for several minutes before changing positions.

Yoga Is Gentler ▶ The old locker-room adage "no pain, no gain" has no place in a yoga class. If participants feel the least bit uncomfortable attempting any movement, they signal the teacher, who works with them individually to modify the stretch so they can perform it comfortably. If that's not possible, they don't do it.

Yoga Involves the Whole Body ▶ Most exercise programs concentrate on the large muscle groups: the arms, legs and abdominals. The typical yoga class works these muscles as well but also spends time flexing the fingers and toes and rolling the eyes, wrists and ankles, thus exercising muscle groups most other fitness programs ignore.

Yoga Works Up a Sweat ▶ But it's by no means as strenuous as aerobics. Participants' heart rates do not reach the aerobic range. After class, participants usually feel more relaxed then tired.

Yoga Is Meditative ▶ While stretching into the various postures—some as simple as looking up at the ceiling, others as challenging as headstands—participants breathe slowly and deeply, which yoga enthusiasts claim not only strengthens the lungs but clears the mind as well.

Yoga American Style

In recent years, the 4,000-year-old Indian art of yoga has become thoroughly naturalized in this country. Classes abound in every major metropolitan area and in many out-of-the-way places. But to many Americans "yoga" still conjures up exotic images of emaciated men in loincloths and turbans contouring themselves into pretzels for no apparent reason.

The fact is, very few yoga devotees attempt contortions, just as very few runners attempt triathlons. The vast majority of regular yoga practitioners stick to simple, straightforward stretches and practice yoga for the simple reason that they like what it does for their bodies, minds and spirits.

"In recent years," says yoga practitioner William E. Connor, M.D., a professor of medicine at Oregon Health Sciences University in Portland, "the emphasis in exercise programs has been on aerobic workouts for cardiovascular fitness. Cardiovascular fitness is certainly worth developing, but aerobic exercise isn't everything. The body also needs workouts that build flexibility, and it's hard to top yoga for flexibility."

As for yoga's purported mental and spiritual benefits, Dr. Connor says, "They're hard to measure, but most people who practice regularly report increased mental clarity and feelings of emotional well-being. Yoga isn't a religion, but some people say it deepens their appreciation of the spiritual side of life."

"As a scientist," says Mary Pullig Schatz, M.D., a pathologist at Centennial Medical Center in Nashville who has practiced yoga for 15 years, "I have problems with the word *spiritual*, because its meaning is unclear. But I can say that yoga helps me feel mentally invigorated."

Yoga as Medicine

These days, some yoga enthusiasts tout the ancient exercise program not only for fun, fitness, flexibility and mental health but also to help manage several chronic medical conditions, including stress, asthma, arthritis, high blood pressure and lower back pain. The medical literature bears them out. In the past decade, medical journals have published more than 100 studies on the health benefits of yoga.

Stress ▶ "Deep breathing and moderate exercise are two fundamentals of many stress-management programs," Dr. Schatz says. "Yoga includes both. Most people who practice regularly usually say it helps them control everyday stresses, tensions and anxieties."

Asthma ▶ Many studies published in such medical journals as the *Journal of Asthma* show that yoga's emphasis on deep breathing, relaxation and muscle tone helps improve lung function, relaxes the respiratory tract and reduces the likelihood of asthma attacks.

Arthritis ▶ Gentle stretching exercises that move sore joints through their full range of motion are a key to managing arthritis. Dr. Connor says yoga stretches and postures encourage range-of-motion movements without unduly stressing arthritic joints.

High Blood Pressure ▶ High blood pressure, medically known as hypertension, is an important risk factor for heart disease and stroke. In addition to blood pressure–lowering drugs, medical authorities recommend controlling hypertension with a combination of stress management and regular moderate exercise. Yoga provides both. In one recent Indian study, 25 people with high blood pressure enrolled in a six-month yoga program in addition to taking standard medications. Yoga decreased their blood pressure below the levels achieved by drug treatment alone and allowed some participants to reduce their medication dosages.

Low Back Pain ▶ Yoga helps strengthen the muscles that support the back vertebrae without subjecting them to the stresses often caused by other forms of exercise, which can aggravate chronic back problems. For their book, *Backache Relief,* coauthors Arthur Klein and Dava Sobel conducted the first national survey asking chronic back pain sufferers how they controlled their pain over the long term. The respondents answered magazine ads, so they were not a random population sample; nonetheless, the survey produced intriguing results.

Yoga won top honors for long-term pain relief. Ninety-six percent of those who performed yoga regularly reported long-term benefits, and none reported yoga making their backs feel any worse. In contrast, only 28 percent of those who relied on chiropractors reported long-term relief, and 11 percent said chiropractic has made them feel worse. It was a back problem that introduced Dr. Schatz to yoga 15 years ago. "I'd tried everything," she recalls, "pain relievers, bed rest, physical therapy, you name it. A friend suggested I try yoga. I viewed it as my last resort before back surgery. It was amazingly therapeutic for me, and I've been doing it ever since."

Of course, yoga is no cure-all. Dr. Connor and Dr. Schatz say people with asthma, arthritis, high blood pressure, back problems and other medical conditions should not throw away their medications or abandon their physicians in favor of yoga classes. "But in addition to regular medical care, yoga can be quite beneficial for

283
∎

many chronic illnesses," Dr. Connor says.

Dr. Connor calls yoga "generally safe" but says some postures aren't for everyone: "Depending on a person's disease or disability, certain poses might cause problems. Headstands can be a problem for people with back, knee or other musculoskeletal problems. But one of yoga's attractions is that, unlike so many other forms of exercise, good teachers can usually adapt the postures to the special needs of people with chronic medical conditions. Yoga is usually a good form of exercise for people with health problems."

Before enrolling in a yoga class (or starting any exercise program), people over 60 or those with disabilities or chronic medical conditions should consult their physicians. In addition, anyone with a medical problem who decides to pursue yoga should confer with the teacher before enrolling to discuss modifying or abstaining from any problematic postures.

The best way to learn yoga, Dr. Schatz says, is to enroll in a class taught by a well-trained teacher you like. "There are many different styles of yoga," she says, "but Iyengar yoga instructors are rigorously trained, not only in the postures themselves, but in adapting them to beginners and to those with disabilities, chronic illnesses or other special needs."

"One thing I like about yoga is that it's completely portable," Dr. Connor says. "You don't need any special clothing, equipment or a gym. All you need is about ten square feet of floor space. I practice ten minutes a day and take an hour-long class once a week. Yoga has improved my body, mind and spirit. No wonder it's been around for thousands of years."

Index

301
■